Sel ▍▌▍▍▌ ɔks:

CW01572730

Quotes of Wisdom

To Live By

Quotes From A Genius,

Autistic, Empath,

And Savant

BRIAN MICHAEL GOOD

Brian Michael Good

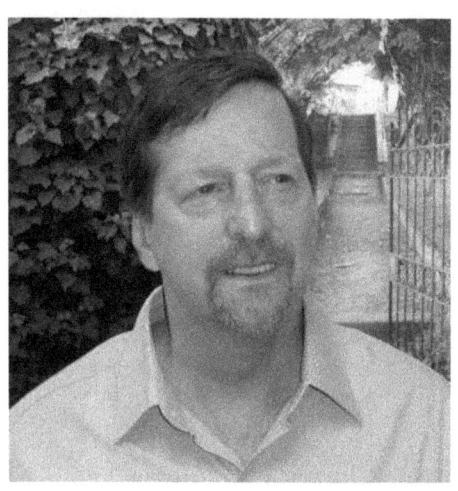

BRIAN MICHAEL GOOD

Spearhead Thinker – Peace Advocate – Author – Writer

Entrepreneur – Genius – Empath – Precious Savant

I am a citizen of the world; not just the citizen of one particular country. I am non-denominational in my belief in God. I am not restricted to any particular or specific religious denomination. That being said; I firmly believe that political, ideological, and religious beliefs that divide our world must be overcome.

Religion and human inequality prevents a more Peaceful World. We must mute the emphasis on religious beliefs that seek to judge others with their tenets and place more emphasis on individually human rights. There are solutions if humankind would listen.

"Mind over matter, if it matters, you will put your mind to it. The mind is capable of solving anything that matters."

— Brian Michael Good

"A book is food for thought… By reading a well written book you will reap pearls of wisdom and have a lifetime of meals."

— Brian Michael Good

Author of "Never Surrender Your Soul, your very essence", "RESET: Control, Alt, Delete", "Quotes of Wisdom to Live By", and "World Peace, Peaceful Worlds, Game Over".

Founder of Nutricare Plus, Tattoo You Organics, and two non-profit startups, Best To Live and Peaceful Worlds, both 501(c)(3) not-for-profit organizations.

Nutricare Plus and Tattoo You Organics market natural health and healing by offering special formulated skin care using the highest quality of herbal, vegan, natural, and organic ingredients.

Peaceful Worlds is a 501(c)(3) not-for-profit organization whose goal is to be an outreach initiative providing answers, information, and provide resources for a more Peaceful World on Earth, our Solar System, and the estimated hundred billion Galaxies in the Universe.

The Best To Live Foundation is a 501(c)(3) not-for-profit organization whose goal is to be an outreach initiative providing answers, information, and provide resources for health needs and overall wellness for anyone who needs to survive emotional, mental, or physical stress.

10% of the "Never Surrender Your Soul" and "RESET: Control, Alt, Delete" and "World Peace Peaceful Worlds Game Over" book's profits will be donated to Peaceful Worlds, a 501(c)(3) not-for-profit if an equal amount is match by the donations of others.

I have lived a life buffeted by character-altering hurricanes. My life storms began in a trauma-filled childhood within my dysfunctional family.

My childhood was filled with tension, excessive discipline, and yelling – at home and at grammar school – contributed to a lower self-esteem and academic performance during my formative developmental years. Yelling and corporal punishment instilled fear in me. I carried such sentiments and emotional trauma with me into adulthood. I accepted the abuse that I allowed others to bestow on me. It took me a lifetime to discover that that I was a Genius, Autistic, Empath, and a Savant.

I survived a childhood of verbal, physical, and sexual abuse; dealt with depression, PTSD, the death of two siblings. A bit further on in life, there was the stigma of being homeless not once, but three times, and bankruptcy two times. I was also diagnosed with a six-pound cancerous tumor that was doubling in size every two months. A suicide attempt in 2003 nearly cost me my life. The death of my best friend, divorce, and the rejection of my only daughter was to follow.

Psychics and people of faith say that we all come back, and some of us come back to teach a lesson. The homeless person on the street has sacrificed their life to teach compassion and tolerance to others. The homeless person, if he or she would know this, might ask, why should I try to improve my life if I came back to suffer to teach this lesson?

The answer is that if one is spiritual, the suffering is only part of the lesson. The most important part is to overcome. We must examine our flaws and try to fix them. Then, in the next chapter of our life, we come back to a better existence.

How can one man encounter so many hurricanes, survive them, learn from them, and then strive to make the world around him a better place? This was the question Brian asked himself that led to this book. I have a deep sense of compassion and empathy for others; social virtues that I value most in my life.

What I have learned from my personal experience can give you hope. You are not alone and you are not forgotten. Your life will improve. Peace and happiness are renewed for those who seek it. I believe that you too will find wisdom in the pearls that have washed ashore as a result of my hurricanes and count yourself a survivor.

Credits

I dedicate "Quotes Of Wisdom To Live By" to my father, John Joseph Good, and my mother, Mary Elizabeth Good. It was hard for my parents to raise eight children. I love you Mom and Dad…

"Nothing of lasting value is given for free; except for the morals, virtues, and lessons taught by our parents."

– Brian Michael Good

Art/Design: "Never Surrender Your Soul, your very essence" and "Quotes of Wisdom to Live By" Front Covers, Best to Live, Big Bang Publishing, and the Tattoo You Organic logos by Alex Polanco

www.AlexPolanco.com

"Perfection on the earthly plain is very rare. Yet, when I gaze upon the artwork for the "Never Surrender Your Soul, your very essence", "RESET: Control, Alt, Delete", "Quotes of Wisdom to Live By", and "World Peace, Peaceful Worlds, Game Over", covers and the "Best To Live" and "Big Bang Publishing" and Tattoo You Organic logos, I see Perfection."

— Brian Michael Good

Design: Back by Daniela Owergoor

www.selfpubbookcovers.com/Daniela

"I love Daniela Owergoor's illustration of the back of the "Quotes of Wisdom to Live By" book."

BRIAN MICHAEL GOOD

Peaceful Worlds

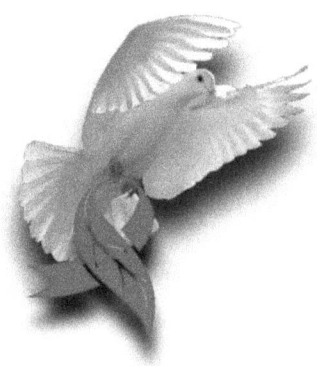

www.facebook.com/PeacefulWorlds

"Striving for a more Peaceful World, one human at a time."

Peaceful Worlds is a 501(c)(3) not-for-profit organization whose goal is to be an outreach initiative providing answers, information, and provide resources for a more Peaceful World on Earth, our Solar System, and the estimated hundred billion Galaxies in the Universe.

Take the "Peaceful Worlds Lemon-Aid Challenge.

We need to talk about lemons, in other words, help create a more Peaceful World by disengaging from mankind's terror. Take the I am Peace… We are Peace... Pledge. We would like you to take the

#PeacefulWorldsLemonAidChallenge as a way to raise money for the Peaceful Worlds non-profit. We challenge you to eat three slices of lemon or donate $10.00 to Peaceful Worlds.

"When life gives you lemons, make lemonade" is a proverbial phrase used to encourage optimism and a can-do attitude in the face of adversity or misfortune. Lemons suggest bitterness, while lemonade is a sweet drink. – Wikipedia

----

Never Surrender to Mankind's Terror, Be a Survivor, SURVIVE one day at a time knowing that no one can defeat the human race. The human race can only defeat themselves.

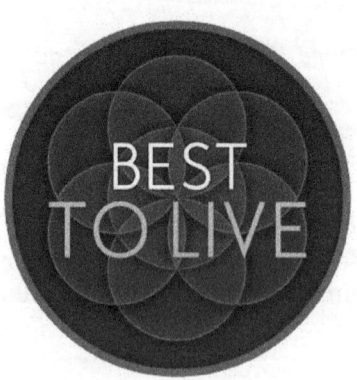

www.BestToLive.org

Best To Live, is a 501(c)(3) non-profit, whose goal is to be an outreach initiative providing answers, information, and provide resources for health needs and overall wellness for anyone who needs to survive emotional, mental, or physical stress.

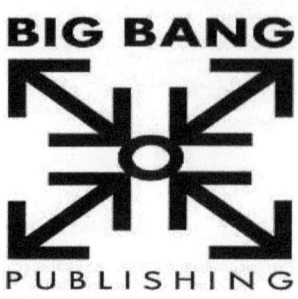

BIG BANG

PUBLISHING

"Quotes Of Wisdom To Live By" can be purchased for educational, business, sales promotions, youth groups, personal growth, self-help, positive thinking, happiness, motivational, success, inspirational, finding your destiny, self-fulfillment use, mental illness, depression, anxiety, or fear. Inquire about a wholesale price from a distributor or from Brian Michael Good, author or Big Bang Publisher at the address, Facebook Messenger or phone number above.

Disclaimer

Content and information contained in "Quotes of Wisdom to Live By is not a substitute for professional medical advice, counseling, diagnosis, or treatment. Nor is it intended to replace a consultation with a qualified medical professional. Never delay or disregard seeking professional medical or mental health advice from your physician or other qualified health provider because of something you have read about in "Quotes of Wisdom to Live By" Brian Michael Good, "Author" and Big Bang Publishing do not diagnose, prescribe or treat anyone medically.

"Quotes of Wisdom to Live By" is designed to provide inspiration to reader's world-wide. It is sold with the understanding that the author and publisher are not engaged to render any type of psychological, legal, financial or any other form of professional advice. The content of each chapter is the sole expression and opinion of the author. No warranties or guarantees are expressed or implied by the author. Neither the publisher nor the individual author shall be liable for any physical, psychological, emotional, financial or commercial damages, including, but not limited to, special, incidental, consequential or other damages. The views and rights of the author and publisher are the same: You are responsible for your own choices, actions, and results.

BRIAN MICHAEL GOOD

Table of Contents

BRIAN MICHAEL GOOD

Introduction

Time is in short supply. Recharge your life with the author's guidance and over 400 quotes thematically arranged in seventy chapters for daily living to encourage and guide you through difficult and challenging times. "Quotes Of Wisdom To Live By" like a 365 day devotional book provides the reader encouragement, comfort, and peace by finding the right words of wisdom at the right time.

As you absorb each quote, you will learn that no one can defeat you; you can only defeat yourself. No one can truly save you. You must save yourself.

Learn how to rise from the ashes of defeat by gaining pearls of wisdom and renewed hope. Open yourself to what I have gleamed from my harsh personal experience.

You are not alone or forgotten. Your life will improve. Peace and happiness are renewed for those who seek it. In picking up this book, you have shown that you want a fulfilling and happy life.

Reap the manna sown into this motivational and inspirational book. Life's most valuable pearls of wisdom that are nourishment for the body, mind, and soul are found in quotation books. There no better gift to another person than the gift of knowledge and understanding derived from wisdom.

"A book of quotes can help change your perspective by allowing you to infuse new activities into your life.

Take action, you will be so happy you did!"

— Brian Michael Good

Abuse

"A woman's adrenaline can overcome her size disadvantage and defeat a man twice her size, but this surge in strength may not be enough if a weapon is used, unless she is trained in self-defense. A woman's emergency hormone adrenaline effect will allow her to lift a car if a loved one is pinned underneath. The "fight or flight" mechanism spurred by adrenaline for primitive women/mothers allowed them to defend their children while the man was away hunting."

— Brian Michael Good

"Having your car keys in your hand with the ignition key extended between two fingers is much better than holding onto your cell phone, which can easily be knocked out of your hand. If you are assaulted… scream out the word "Fire" not "Rape". People respond better to the word 'fire' because it may affect their safety. If all else fails sexual predators love to be in control. If you grab their privates, they may be startled enough for you to escape."

— Brian Michael Good

"Self-defense should be taught to all children so they can combat rape, sexual abuse, and physical assault, which could happen to anyone. The confidence gained in the ability to defend oneself should never be overlooked in any person's development."

— Brian Michael Good

"Never put your self-esteem in the hands of an abuser… by listening to them."

— Brian Michael Good

"The abuse is often forgiven as time heals, it should never be forgotten; otherwise we will not learn from the past for whatever we chose to forget will be repeated."

— Brian Michael Good

"The evil in your life is the abuse you allow others to bestow on you. So, if you are a survivor like me, and others like me, just be fearless. It might be the only way to save you from fear. Fear can consume you and spit you out dead."

— Brian Michael Good

"My childhood was filled with tension, excessive discipline, and yelling – at home and at grammar school – each contributed to a lower self-esteem and academic performance during my formative developmental years. Yelling and corporal punishment instilled fear in me. I carried such sentiments and emotional trauma with me into adulthood."

— Brian Michael Good

"I accepted the abuse that I allowed others to bestow on me. It took me a lifetime to discover that people do not scar or give you pain. It was my acceptance of their mistreatment. I blame myself for not being able to heal from the hurt and the scars that I now realize were self-inflicted. I found that self-pity was one of my greatest weaknesses. Self-pity doesn't do anyone any good. We are all much stronger than we initially think when something bad happens in our life."

— Brian Michael Good

"I started by taking an abuse course (not court ordered – my choice – you know – free will). After my suicide attempt I took and passed an anger management course. These self-help programs helped me to become a better person."

— Brian Michael Good

"Children seldom react well to the harsh tone of your voice, by placing your hand over their mouth, by pulling them by their hands, or by spanking them. Positive reinforcement will help your children to develop a positive self-esteem. Positive reinforcement works far better than any form of discipline that causes excessive fear or anxiety in your child's development."

— Brian Michael Good

"Forgiving is not forgetting; it's actually remembering by not becoming an abuser; by using your free will not to hit back with anger, hatred, or revenge. It's an opportunity for a new beginning, a second chance, a learning experience by not allowing anyone to hurt or abuse you again."

— Brian Michael Good

"You must find a way to live even if you suffer from shunning, teasing, gossiping, bullying, shaming, child abuse, sexual abuse, verbal and/or physical abuse. You are the one who is responsible for your own life and the decisions you make."

— Brian Michael Good

"Sorry means nothing if a person takes no future action to avoid being sorry again."

— Brian Michael Good

"Learn to defend yourself. Take a defense course. You have the right to defend your ground but why take the chance of going to jail if you use excessive force."

— Brian Michael Good

Acceptance

\-

"Acceptance is letting go of the past to get ahead in the present"

— Brian Michael Good

\-

"Acceptance is a gift that helps you to skip forward and live in the present."

— Brian Michael Good

\-

"Sometimes you meet someone and you can skip forward because of the greeting, the acceptance, and the goodbye"

— Brian Michael Good

\-

"Take responsibility for the decisions that you have made in the past that have bought you to where you are in life."

— Brian Michael Good

\-

"Only you as an individual can improve the way you are viewed. It begins with how you view yourself. You are in control of how you are perceived by others by realizing that your self-esteem should not be connected with the acceptance of others."

— Brian Michael Good

\-

"How you view yourself should be far more important than what others think of you. Accepting yourself the way you are is the best gift you can give yourself. You are much better than you think you are."

— Brian Michael Good

"Everyone needs a chance to be fulfilled with acceptance, which is the impetus to heal old wounds."

— Brian Michael Good

"Waiting was the hardest part, and finally one person and the acceptance among strangers pushed me over the fence totally into the present."

— Brian Michael Good

"Talking to yourself once in a blue moon is acceptable. Arguing with yourself is not acceptable.

So, why are you still in denial?"

— Brian Michael Good

"Acceptance and forgiveness will help you heal and sets us free. Say these words and be healed. The past is forgiven. You have the key; just unlock the chain. You are free. It is the only way to be free, find peace and happiness. It is a choice?"

— Brian Michael Good

"When you meet another person or when two or more are gathered you will have the opportunity to create the gift of acceptance, the epitome of what humanity should be! The higher you raise yourself in the better treatment of others, the better view you will have of the future."

— Brian Michael Good

"Say hello to a stranger. They will greet you with acceptance and a smile almost every time."

— Brian Michael Good

"Accepting yourself the way you are is the secret to happiness and finding peace in your life. You can allow your experiences to destroy you or redefine you. Forget about whom you were; accept who you are, and who you can be.

That is a choice!"

— Brian Michael Good

"How to improve your physical, emotional or mental well-being.

You need to change your perspective in layers of acceptance and understanding. We all have the power within us to change. We must Reset from the inside out. One day at a time. Exercise, Diet, and finding your passion help us to change.

Change has always been part of human survival."

— Brian Michael Good

"Just do the very best you can do… Create a fresh attitude by changing your perspective; the way you think will go a long way in making you happy. Acceptance is the key. To forgive is to let GO.

You must RESET:

You are in: CONTROL
Change your perspective: ALT
Forget the past: DELETE."

— Brian Michael Good

Ageing

"We are taught to nurture the health of our body, mind, and soul; often they are neglected. While our health declines as each year passes, we value our soul more knowing that it is all that will remain."

— Brian Michael Good

"If you are prepared to enter the afterlife, the day you die should be a bigger celebration than the day you are born."

— Brian Michael Good

"The clock's ticking… The longer you wait to change your life the harder it becomes to implement change. Sixty years old is mid-life if you consider that a healthy person with modern medical care might live to one hundred twenty. So what are you waiting for? Do something with your life."

— Brian Michael Good

Anger

"The best fight won is the fight not fought."

— Brian Michael Good

"Rather than listening to the person with anger in their voice, empower yourself by listening to your inner voice of reason."

— Brian Michael Good

"Forgiving is not forgetting; it's actually remembering by not becoming an abuser; yet, using your free will not to hit back with anger or revenge. It's an opportunity for a new beginning, a second chance, a learning experience by not allowing anyone to hurt or abuse you again."

— Brian Michael Good

Anxiety

"Most of us live our lives in the proactive, reactive, or passive mode. When you are proactive you tend to be positive and prepare for what could happen. When you are reactive you tend to respond when something is about to happen.

A proactive approach can result in a better opportunity for control and fulfillment whereas the reactive mode can result in more stress that can make any problem even more difficult to solve which may lead to failure. A passive life is as if you never lived at all."

— Brian Michael Good

"When you remember the past too much you don't heal and this can lead to depression. When you try to view the future too much, it can cause anxiety. But when you live in the Now; it makes you feel right; glad to be living in the moment."

— Brian Michael Good

"Just like water, wind, waves, and ice are the agents of erosion of our beaches that bring changes to our shorelines; fear, anxiety, and depression are the agents of erosion of our hope that bring changes to our mental, physical or spiritual health.

— Brian Michael Good

"Fear, anxiety, and depression decreases in exact proportion to your increase in hope."

— Brian Michael Good

"You will not to be held captive by fear, anxiety, or depression."

— Brian Michael Good

"Children seldom react well to the harsh tone of your voice, by placing your hand over their mouth, by pulling them by their hands, or by spanking them. Positive reinforcement will help your children to develop a positive self-esteem. Positive reinforcement works far better than any form of discipline that causes excessive fear or anxiety in your child's development."

— Brian Michael Good

Attitude

"Your attitude affects your self-esteem and how you are viewed by others"

— Brian Michael Good

"Only you can improve the way you view yourself and how you are perceived by others. You can affect change in your self-esteem and improve the way you view yourself with a positive mental attitude."

— Brian Michael Good

"Challenges, hardships, and obstacles are part of what life's journey is all about. You are not always in control of what happens to you, but you are in control how you react to it. You can allow your experiences to destroy you or redefine you."

— Brian Michael Good

"Never let your attitude be the reason for your failure."

— Brian Michael Good

"A positive attitude influences our behavior and dictates a successful approach."

— Brian Michael Good

"I will overcome… are the three most powerful words you can think out loud. Our thoughts often become our reality."

— Brian Michael Good

"No one can defeat you. You can only defeat yourself. No one can truly save you. You can only save yourself. It's a choice."

— Brian Michael Good

"Being more positive can help heal life's disappointments. Your perception of what happens in your life and having realistic expectations creates a positive influence in your life."

— Brian Michael Good

"A person who navigates life's challenges, hardships, and obstacles with stern resolve is able to sail in all winds."

— Brian Michael Good

"Don't be fearful of the future. Own it by allowing yourself to absorb only the positive energy of the people you choose to surround yourself in your new life instead of the negative energy of the old crowd."

— Brian Michael Good

I voted...

"It is not whether I think that my vote counts in any election. What matters is that my vote counts to me."

— Brian Michael Good

"Just do the very best you can do. Create a fresh attitude by changing your perspective; the way you think will go a long way in making you happy. Acceptance is the key. To forgive is to let GO.

You must RESET:

You are in: CONTROL
Change your perspective: ALT
Forget the past: DELETE."

— Brian Michael Good

Beauty

"There is more beauty in someone who is humble than someone who sees themselves as perfect."

— Brian Michael Good

"If you are independent, strong, weak, confident, intelligent, average, size, shape, old-fashioned, athletic, fashionable, or style less, these attributes or your size, shape, or attire should not diminish your femininity/beauty/essence, nor should your femininity/beauty/essence diminish your equality. I believe in the equalism movement for all humans, absence of required roles, labels, or behaviors that gender may require."

— Brian Michael Good

"You are much better than you think you are and you are more beautiful/handsome than you think you are."

— Brian Michael Good

"Beauty on this earthly plane is often short lived... A beautiful heart and soul will last an eternity."

— Brian Michael Good

Belief

"The most important decision you will make in your life is what you choose for your beliefs since they have everything to do with how you live."

— Brian Michael Good

"I believe that the best defense against – giving up your soul – your very essence – is your choice of a belief system based on faith, hope, knowledge, reason, and logic."

— Brian Michael Good

"Eternal life has just as much to do with what we do right as what we do wrong."

— Brian Michael Good

"Do you believe because you understand, or do you understand because you believe?"

— Brian Michael Good

"Are we that gullible or should we call the story of how Adam and Eve were created as told in "The Book of Genesis" mind control?"

— Brian Michael Good

"Religion is often written with a controlled message, a form of mind control."

— Brian Michael Good

"You should nurture your belief system as a mother nurtures an infant. It is best to choose a belief system that allows you to be fair-minded and even-handed. Be aware you may lose your visa based on the belief system you choose, making your ticket to the afterlife with your soul unable to reach your desired destination."

— Brian Michael Good

"Modern society sets the benchmark for eternal life far lower than it has ever truly been because our morals have lapsed and yet we still want a feel-good comfort about death and the afterlife even though we have morally failed. The moment you feel you are saved, it may put you in a comfort zone where you forfeit your ticket to the afterlife by surrendering your soul with complacency."

— Brian Michael Good

"Eighty percent of the people on our planet have dark skin? If eighty percent of the people on our planet have dark skin and Adam and Eve come from Africa, then I surmise that Adam and Eve had dark skin. I conclude that a dark Adam and Eve were created in Africa, substantiated by logic, science, reason, and faith. That's right Adam and Eve were dark; as dark as my large two inch birthmark, a Café au lait spot, and freckles; remnants of the dark seed."

— Brian Michael Good

"Science has proven with DNA testing that all races have developed from Africa. Darker humans became white when they moved to the northern climates of Europe. They lived in the mountains and ate a different diet than in Africa. Humans in India had a lot of spice and different food in their diet. In Asia, their diet was mostly fish, vegetables, and less meat. Humans adapted to their different environments all over our planet. Aborigines from Australia came from Africa over sixty thousand years ago and they are dark from the original human seed."

— Brian Michael Good

"One to four percent of the DNA of the extinct Neanderthals and up to five percent Siberian DNA (Asians) is found in the DNA of billions of present day humans except for two villages in Africa who are 100% human. The ancestors of these two villages did not interbreed with Neanderthals or the Siberians. Dark skinned humans have a higher level of melanin in their skin. As dark skinned humans moved out of Africa into northern Europe, they lost the amount of melanin in their skin from the lack of sunlight. Each generation inherited lighter skin. Diet, climate, and the environment influenced the formation of different human races."

— Brian Michael Good

"Adam might need a touch up with darker skin color in the Sistine Chapel ceiling representation of the Christian Bible of Faith's Genesis. It does not make sense that Adam is painted white when eighty percent people living on the planet Earth have dark skin.

Again, mind control at its best. It is no longer a white man's world anymore. When it comes to the skin color of humans, it was never the white man's world."

— Brian Michael Good

First Commandment: I am the Lord, your God.

Is Jesus God? God is not Jesus.

Jesus was not born yet when the Ten Commandments were created.

Who is Weshemehe? [God]

Judaism, Hinduism, Christianity states that God is omnipresent; it might be referenced in Islam, Quran 2:115. If God is present everywhere (in all places at all times), then God is part of every atom in the universe. If the universe is God. Therefore, God does not have a gender.

If God does not have a gender, I choose to use the word Weshemehe (We-she-me-he), my own English name for God, who represents all genders. More importantly, it means more than just the male gender as the word God denotes to many of us.

Weshemehe means we are all part of the universe and part of Weshemehe. Weshemehe is the entire universe whereas Jesus is a bigger part of Weshemehe and the universe than the rest of us but not omnipresent (everywhere – in all places at all times) like Weshemehe.

Jesus said, "For where two or three are gathered together in my name, there am I in the midst of them." – Matthew 18:20, KJV

Pope Francis has stated that Evolution and the Big Bang Theory are real. The Big Bang was initiated by Weshemehe in order to create the universe and share life with all of us. Weshemehe, being omnipresent, is part of the reason why Weshemehe can control anything at any moment, and how you can have a personal relationship with Weshemehe.

Second Commandment: Thou shall bring no false idols before me.

"Christians should make a note of these facts:

God never left the throne, Jesus sits to the right of God, Jesus talked to God while on Earth, Jesus respects his Father as I respect my Father, and Jesus praises God, as I praise God.

God is not Jesus, Jesus is son of God, and Holy Spirit is son of God.

No man or woman can be God for God is the entire Universe.

Jesus and the Holy Spirit are instruments of God and derived their power and miracles only from God's Grace."

— Brian Michael Good

"It would be wise not break the First and Second Commandments by putting Jesus or the Holy Spirit in front of God. For God is Good."

— Brian Michael Good

"Be forewarned... God's judgement and vengeance is close at hand...

Too many humans have forsaken God and the 10 Commandments."

— Brian Michael Good

"I do not believe vaccinations cause autism. I was born with autism. I had my own language consisting of repetitive words that only my mother understood. I was fortunate to have been raised in a family of 8 children, I was forced to grow into a hundred percent functioning adult from the constant interaction with my many siblings. I am a Genius, Empath, and Precious Savant with Asperger's Syndrome; which use to be on the autistic spectrum until a few years ago.

I believe that there are more autistic children born because some of them will help save humanity... If you can find their passion, there is a chance you will discover how special they truly are...They might be a Genius, Empath or Savant... Maybe all three."

— Brian Michael Good

Business

\-----------------------------

"Before you can be successful you must have the right perspective and mindset. Seize the day and Recharge your life."

— Brian Michael Good

\-----------------------------

"Working is a pleasure. When providing for the ones you love... is your happiness."

— Brian Michael Good

\-----------------------------

"Without collaboration we could never make the strides of progress."

— Brian Michael Good

\-----------------------------

"No human is an island if they want to successful."

— Brian Michael Good

\-----------------------------

"2017 will be my year... I have risen from the ashes of defeat...

I was 30 minutes from death on October 23, 2003 from my near death experience.

I never got my "Big Break" or took full advantage of someone who discovered me and the rest was easy.

So I have decided that I need to take it upon myself to Break Out Big."

— Brian Michael Good

"Seven out of ten people do not enjoy their vocation. Most of the time people find their first couple of jobs by circumstance or chance rather than creating a plan based on their passion. Going to college for four years and getting a degree or working in a trade may increase your income potential an additional four hundred dollars a week more than a person with a high school degree over the course of your career."

— Brian Michael Good

"Value the passion you have for your life's work more than you value material gain."

— Brian Michael Good

"Great things come from people who are not afraid to risk making others around them feel uncomfortable with their futuristic vision."

— Brian Michael Good

"Authority, control, and wealth come with great responsibility. The Creator expects major shareholders, management and business owners to pay honest wages for an honest day's work. Greed does not give you any reward in the afterlife. You have already taken more than your fair share."

— Brian Michael Good

"If you never venture out of your comfort zone and put your idea into action. Another person surely will."

— Brian Michael Good

"The average woman does eighty percent of the buying, is more intelligent, better at multi-tasking, budgeting, prioritizing than the average man. Forty-two percent of the heads of family households are woman and many of them have a full time job. Women in the USA earn approximately seventy-seven percent of what a man earns for the same jobs.

If we change our perception, we may discover that the pendulum should swing to the opposite direction where men earn seventy-seven percent of what women earn.

Now, that's good karma."

— Brian Michael Good

"Individual humans work together with other individual humans but the human race does not work together with nature and the Creator if the human race buys products whose raw materials damage the environment (the Creator's gift) and the wars where humans participate and started/influenced by big business and the wealthy destroy innocent lives."

— Brian Michael Good

"Every endeavor in life is not about the odds of success but about your belief, your passion, and your indomitable will."

— Brian Michael Good

Change

"You should effect change when it comes to your emotional, mental, physical, or spiritual health."

— Brian Michael Good

"You must get out of comfort zone if you are ever going to change."

— Brian Michael Good

Forget about whom you were; accept who you are, and who you can be.

That is a choice!"

— Brian Michael Good

"You can change the future only by implementing change in the present."

— Brian Michael Good

"Without change you will likely fail. If you fail you must change."

— Brian Michael Good

"Try not to create your own misery by staying with the old you, by not having an awakening that motivates you to change. Sometimes in order to re-invent yourself you need to be like a caterpillar and be alone for a while in order to turn into a butterfly."

— Brian Michael Good

"You must strive to act as the person you would like to become, as an actor would become the persona of the character of a play or movie. It takes at least thirteen weeks before you transition/change into a new person. You must believe that you are the "new you" before other people perceive "you" as this "new you.""

— Brian Michael Good

"The clock's ticking… The longer you wait to change your life the harder it becomes to implement change. Sixty years old is mid-life if you consider that a healthy person with modern medical care might live to one hundred twenty. So what are you waiting for? Do something with your life."

— Brian Michael Good

"It has been said that in a lifetime we live many lives. If you don't like your life begin your next life within your present life by implementing change in the present."

— Brian Michael Good

"Plan a change. Do something different in your life — move out of your comfort zone. What is most important is the foundation, a step by step outline of your plan that will encourage you to do something different outside your comfort zone. Your plan will likely fail without a step by step outline, the change may not happen if you don't plan or follow through with your plan to venture out of your comfort zone."

— Brian Michael Good

"Think out of box, do things differently, travel, meet people. Changing the way you think is part of survival. Change your daily life's activities and you will change your life."

— Brian Michael Good

"How to improve your physical, emotional or mental well-being.

You need to change your perspective in layers of acceptance and understanding. We all have the power within us to change. We must Reset from the inside out. One day at a time. Exercise, Diet, and finding your passion help us to change.

Change has always been part of human survival."

— Brian Michael Good

"Your life can change without notice; in just seconds that could change your life's course forever… only if you let it. Nearly everything can be fixed. A choice."

— Brian Michael Good

BRIAN MICHAEL GOOD

Change the World

"Don't wait until the later years of your life to realize that you could've been an integral part of the impetus of change that could have indeed changed the world."

— Brian Michael Good

"If you do not try to change your world, your world will change you."

— Brian Michael Good

"Change your world peacefully or your world will change you. You are either the <u>hammer</u> — writer — supplier — leader — speaker or the <u>nail</u> — reader — consumer — follower — audience. The hammer and the nail were designed to build the world together and create good not to destroy. Become the positive hammer and nail of change that you would like to see in the world. Build a better world."

— Brian Michael Good

"Spirituality will be accepted as the universal standard in our world if the human species is to survive. Spirituality marks a turning point in the world's religious thinking; that the afterlife is open to anyone regardless of his or her religious belief. Unconditional acceptance of religious differences in our society that are derived from cultural differences in our world."

— Brian Michael Good

"You don't think that God doesn't know every nuclear launch code in the world!

What are you thinking?

You are making it so easy for God to commence Game Over — Burnt Toast — Nuclear War — Armageddon that we are racing toward is… 100% Guaranteed."

— Brian Michael Good

Compassion

"Have kindness, compassion, and empathy towards others and the natural environment."

— Brian Michael Good

"I have a deep sense of compassion and empathy for others; social virtues that I value most in my life."

— Brian Michael Good

"Without the help of strangers, my recovery from cancer and suicide attempt would have been quite difficult."

— Brian Michael Good

"Help someone in need with kindness including yourself."

— Brian Michael Good

"Psychics and people of faith say that we all come back, and some of us come back to teach a lesson. The homeless person on the street has sacrificed their life to teach compassion and tolerance to others. The homeless person, if he or she would know this, might ask, why should I try to improve my life if I came back to suffer to teach this lesson? The answer is that if one is spiritual, the suffering is only part of the lesson. The most important part is to overcome. We must examine our flaws and try to fix them. Then, in the next chapter of our life, we come back to a better existence."

— Brian Michael Good

Confidence

"Self-defense should be taught to all children so they can combat rape, sexual abuse, and physical assault, which could happen to anyone. The confidence gained in the ability to defend oneself should never be overlooked in any person's development."

— Brian Michael Good

"You are much better than you think you are and you are more beautiful/handsome than you think you are."

— Brian Michael Good

"You are in control of how you are perceived by others by realizing that your self-esteem and confidence should not be connected with the acceptance of others."

— Brian Michael Good

"A person with a positive and confident self-image holds his head up high and is self-aware of their surroundings whereas a person with a low self-esteem or a poor self-image looks away from others or looks down with their head bowed which causes drooping shoulders."

— Brian Michael Good

"Think of a happy thought or something that you are good at that allows you to walk in a confident manner with a smile. Look straight ahead as you walk, make eye contact whenever you talk or pass someone in the school hallways."

— Brian Michael Good

"How you make eye contact with someone reveals a lot about your confidence and self-esteem."

— Brian Michael Good

Control

"All we can really do or control is living in the moment."

— Brian Michael Good

"History is often written with a controlled message, a form of mind control."

— Brian Michael Good

"Find a man/woman/partner that will appreciate everything about you who won't try to change you or control your free will."

— Brian Michael Good

"Change your perspective with less mind control so you can live a hopeful life that creates a path with less fear."

— Brian Michael Good

"A big part of dealing with depression is realizing that you are in control of your own happiness."

— Brian Michael Good

"If you control your body, emotions, and desires, you will be in control of the family finances in your future marriage/relationship."

— Brian Michael Good

"How you manage your expectations is the secret to happiness and finding peace in your life. Peace and happiness are renewed for those who seek it. Take control of your life and be a survivor. Forget about whom you were; accept who you are, and who you can be.

That is a choice!"

— Brian Michael Good

"Most of us live our lives in the proactive, reactive, or passive mode. When you are proactive you tend to be positive and prepare for what could happen. When you are reactive you tend to respond when something is about to happen.

A proactive approach can result in a better opportunity for control and fulfillment whereas the reactive mode can result in more stress that can make any problem even more difficult to solve which may lead to failure. A passive life is as if you never lived at all."

— Brian Michael Good

"Your children are born with free will. You cannot control their free will without consequences. You are meant to be their guides."

— Brian Michael Good

"If you decide to walk the path of life in complete control of your free will you must resist mind control by adopting a knowledge or faith belief system that is aided with logic and facts."

— Brian Michael Good

"Do not attempt to control anyone's free will."

— Brian Michael Good

"If you want to control your lover then do not even think of controlling them. When you do not try to control your partner in a relationship, then you are in control and your partner will always be at your side as your best friend. You will receive far more love and respect than a person who wants control in a relationship."

— Brian Michael Good

"A person whose thoughts are exercised with free will has much more clarity than the thoughts of those who readily accept mind control."

— Brian Michael Good

"Choose to begin to change one day at a time, tiny steps where you position yourself in a steady motion of happiness and tranquility instead of allowing yourself to be hashed around beyond your control."

— Brian Michael Good

"Authority, control, and wealth come with great responsibility. The Creator expects major shareholders, management, and business owners to pay honest wages for an honest day's work. Greed does not give you any reward in the afterlife. You have already taken more than your fair share."

— Brian Michael Good

Coping

Get enough sleep

Go for a walk – Get some sunlight

Develop Friendships

Watch your diet

Change your daily routine

Play some good music and chill for awhile

Exercise, Forgiving, Spirituality

Meditation, Journaling, Limit Setting

Visualization, Goal Setting

"Help someone in need with kindness including yourself."

— Brian Michael Good

"Talking to yourself once in a blue moon is acceptable. Arguing with yourself is not acceptable.

So, why are you still in denial?"

— Brian Michael Good

"Songs will never grow old when they are done by great performers. Play some good music and enjoy a comfortable chill by listening to your favorite music. A great coping skill."

— Brian Michael Good

"Develop a way to clear your head… Just say a positive phrase silently or out loud by repeating it to yourself until it clears your head."

— Brian Michael Good

"Find me and you will find yourself."

— Brian Michael Good

"Acceptance: Let go of the past to get ahead in the present."

— Brian Michael Good

"Do not dwell on problems in which you cannot effect any change."

— Brian Michael Good

"Develop a way to clear your head… Just say the words cancel – clear."

— Brian Michael Good

"Everyone deserves a "Me" day without any guilt or regret... Relax and enjoy a day off."

— Brian Michael Good

Courage

"Life's journey often requires great courage to overcome our greatest fears."

— Brian Michael Good

"It takes courage to be able to deal with life's sudden changes. You may not fully recover, but you can adapt. The battle is often won by finding a source of hope that will push you forward."

— Brian Michael Good

"It takes courage to break the chain reaction cycles we get into... It like a whirlpool, there seems to be no way out."

— Brian Michael Good

Death

"Do not kill emotionally, mentally, physically, or spiritually."

— Brian Michael Good

"Except for my suicide attempt, each time I faced death; I knew I wanted to live."

— Brian Michael Good

"Suicide is often referred to as a permanent solution to a temporary problem."

— Brian Michael Good

"Death by suicide might include any irresponsible, dangerous, or reckless behavior that causes your premature death; except for dangerous situations, someone may encounter in the military, public service, occupation, sports activity, or an unavoidable accident."

— Brian Michael Good

"I am very blessed to be alive and to be a survivor of many near death experiences."

— Brian Michael Good

"Illicit drug abuse, drunk driving, binge drinking, and overdosing on prescription drugs is playing Russian roulette. In each case you knew there was a chance that the shot you were about to take could cause your death.

It was your decision to insert the needle into your body and take the shot of drugs that killed you. It was your choice to shoot shots of alcohol and the binge drinking that lead to your drunk driving death.

It was your decision to take more than the normal dose of prescription drugs or by taking a combination of different drugs without reading the instructions – disclaimers – that caused you die from your drug overdose. Just like it was your decision to place the muzzle against your head and pull the trigger of the gun that shot the bullet that killed you. In each case you took your life and died by suicide."

— Brian Michael Good

"My near death experience from my self-induced drug overdose should have killed me and wiped my brain clean like reformatting a hard drive on your computer. My life and brain were spared?"

— Brian Michael Good

"Why would you kill yourself when there are an infinite number of possible alternatives and positive outcomes?"

— Brian Michael Good

"I ask you with all my heart for you to reconsider… killing yourself? I wanted to live after my suicide attempt when I awoke from my coma two and one half days later."

— Brian Michael Good

"If you are prepared to enter the afterlife, the day you die should be a bigger celebration than the day you are born."

— Brian Michael Good

"I have no doubt I should be dead from my near-fatal suicide attempt, my cancer, and other times when I was an inch from death. I thought my life would be over when I tried to die by suicide.

Little did I know that my life was just beginning. I have everything to live for… A Choice…

We-she-me-he (the Creator) of second chances I am safe, for the moment at least."

The Creator works in mysterious ways."

— Brian Michael Good

"I am a survivor. I now respect the gift that The Creator has given all of us: life. I am very grateful to be alive."

— Brian Michael Good

Denial

"Talking to yourself once in a blue moon is acceptable. Arguing with yourself is not acceptable.

So, why are you still in denial?"

— Brian Michael Good

"It took this self-induced hurricane; my suicide attempt, when I did not heed the advice given to me to evacuate the coast by properly dealing with personal issues including mental health, eviction, taxes, unemployment, and a failed marriage, which lead to three months of rehab for my twisted foot from my drug overdose, then eight months of homelessness. Ironically, these were the first steps to the road of recovery."

— Brian Michael Good

Depression

"You will not to be held captive by fear, anxiety or depression."

— Brian Michael Good

"A big part of dealing with depression is realizing that you are in control of your own happiness."

— Brian Michael Good

"Some of us will experience some form of mental illness in their lifetime… I rather have depression that can be treated with a pill and my free will to conquer it; than have a physical illness that results in my demise because no matter what I did I could not conquer it."

— Brian Michael Good

"Depression is like a rip tide current that never ends. If you try to swim back to shore, your efforts will be futile and it will only tire you out and make it that much more difficult for you to survive. To escape depression just like the rip tide current you need to swim sideways or seek help; by allowing a lifeguard… 800-273-TALK (8255) or medicine carry you to calmer waters."

— Brian Michael Good

"Fear, anxiety, and depression decreases in exact proportion to your increase in hope."

— Brian Michael Good

"We are powerless when the wind, water, waves, and ice are the agents of the erosion of our beaches that brings changes to our shorelines. We have the power to do something when we allow fear, anxiety or depression to be the agents of the erosion of our hope that affects our emotional, mental, physical or spiritual health. A choice."

— Brian Michael Good

"Life is not only precious but living your life in a developed country is a privileged life compared to living your life in a third world country. There is always someone in the world that would be willing to take your place and fight your fight. They will gladly learn to live with your pain, adapt to your depression, overcome your fears; not die by suicide and live the rest of your life at peace. This is why death by suicide is an unforgivable act because there are so many others who would love to have your life."

— Brian Michael Good

"Suicidal thoughts can last for days, weeks, months or even years. I want you to know that you are not alone in your experience. The answers to your questions are all around you. Sometimes, all it takes is to admit to yourself that you need help to effect a positive change when it comes to your mental, physical, emotional or spiritual health. Call 800-273-TALK (8255) if you need a friend to lean on."

— Brian Michael Good

"There will never be enough breath in your lungs to sustain the depths of your despair; just like the depths of the ocean cannot be sustained indefinitely without being resupplied with fresh air. In both cases you will not survive unless you take the necessary action needed before your final breath. Come up for air by going for a walk and just breathe."

— Brian Michael Good

Desire

"Think about a car not having ample petro/gas to start the engine, as the body not getting the proper nutrition, preventing the driver from arriving at their desired destination.

An engaged mind likewise cannot develop the knowledge base on life skills that will be needed to achieve upward mobility."

— Brian Michael Good

"Be aware you may lose your visa based on the belief system you choose, making your ticket to the afterlife with your soul unable to reach your desired destination."

— Brian Michael Good

"Guide your children so they can realize their own separate dream. Lead them in the right direction only means guidance, not pushing them against their will into a school, a sport, a high school, a social group, a college, or leading them on a career path where they will lack the passion or desire to excel."

— Brian Michael Good

"If you control your body, emotions, and desires, you will be in control of the finances in your future marriage/relationship."

— Brian Michael Good

BRIAN MICHAEL GOOD

Despair

"There will never be enough breath in your lungs to sustain the depths of your despair; just like the depths of the ocean cannot be sustained indefinitely without being resupplied with fresh air. In both cases you will not survive unless you take the necessary action needed before your final breath. Come up for air by going for a walk and just breathe."

— Brian Michael Good

"You can do all the right things and still have bad results. Bad things happen to good people and sometimes bad things happen for a reason. Someday, in your future, there is going to be a better tomorrow. Know that things will get better."

— Brian Michael Good

"How you manage your expectations is the secret to happiness and finding peace in your life. Peace and happiness are renewed for those who seek it. Take control of your life and be a survivor. Forget about whom you were; accept who you are, and who you can be.

That is a choice!"

— Brian Michael Good

"Changes or events that happen in your life can be fixed or healed with a positive mental attitude. A choice. But when your life is over;

it never comes back and you'll never know you could have made it to where you once thought was impossible. Again, a choice."

— Brian Michael Good

"Stop feeling sorry for yourself because only you can save yourself. Pick yourself up, go take a walk, meet a new friend, or ask someone out on a date. Meet a new friend that will make you laugh."

— Brian Michael Good

"Do not judge your lot in life and do not over judge yourself. Do not feel sorry for yourself. Stop whining. Do not self-pity. Life can always be worse than it is. Nothing is the end of the world. There is always a way to fix it."

— Brian Michael Good

Destiny and Life

"Six weeks after conception, the nervous system of the developing brain of a fetus is able to send out impulses to control its body functions and movements. Since the lack of brain activity is the accepted as the sign of death in the medical community and accepted by many people of faith. It might be safe to say that the beginning of brain activity is a definitive sign of life.

The heart of a fetus first begins to beat at three weeks, about 18 days after conception. I believe that life begins when the heart of the fetus starts to beat since there has been one medical case where a child was born without a brain and lived for twelve years with a beating heart."

— Brian Michael Good

"Each person's destiny is unique, some are destined to be great; some are destined to inspire greatness and change in others."

— Brian Michael Good

"Your life can change without notice; in just seconds that could change your life's course forever… only if you let it. Nearly everything can be fixed. A choice."

— Brian Michael Good

"Integrity, Honor, Trust, Loyalty, Respect, Reputation. These values should be nurtured as a mother cares for an infant. Without the proper attention, all of these values can be lost from one careless decision."

— Brian Michael Good

"Sometimes the hand that life has dealt us is because of the decisions and actions we have made. We realize we dealt the hand ourselves."

— Brian Michael Good

"Meeting your destiny doesn't happen without a plan, a plan doesn't happen without a purpose, a purpose doesn't happen without finding your passion, a passion isn't discovered without the pursuit of activities that you enjoy."

— Brian Michael Good

"Never put your destiny in the hands of a naysayer… by listening to them."

— Brian Michael Good

"Finding your destiny has much to do with finding out what makes you happy. You need to take the necessary steps to put your life on the right course to find your passion and achieve your destiny. Choose a passion you enjoy doing; so even if do not meet your destiny you will be happy with your life. Always have a backup plan. You may find that your hobby is the passion that becomes your destiny."

— Brian Michael Good

"The only thing you will truly regret in your life is who you could have been. Life will always be what you make of it. Forget about whom you were; accept who you are, and who you can be.

That is a choice!"

— Brian Michael Good

"Find a purpose for your life and you will do extraordinary things.

You are in center of your happiness when you pursue your passion.

When you pursue your passion, you are the master of your environment.

When you are the master of your environment you often meet your destiny."

— Brian Michael Good

"Life's experiences are not woven with a constant thread; Life in our world is constantly changing. We must repurpose what we have endured and the lessons we have learned; creating a renewed sense of hope. Life is what it is. The question is… What are you willing to do to change your life?"

— Brian Michael Good

"Mind over matter, if it matters, you will put your mind to it. The mind is capable of solving anything that matters."

— Brian Michael Good

"Tomorrow is full of promise if you prepare for today."

— Brian Michael Good

"Every endeavor in life is not about the odds of success but about your passion, your belief, and your indomitable will."

— Brian Michael Good

"How you play the hand that life has dealt you will define your human spirit. Do not judge your lot in life and do not over judge yourself. Do not feel sorry for yourself. Stop whining and have no self-pity. Nothing is the end of the world. Life can always be worse than it is. There is always a way to fix it."

— Brian Michael Good

"Great things come from people who are not afraid to risk making others around them feel uncomfortable with their futuristic vision."

— Brian Michael Good

"Change your world peacefully or your world will change you. You are either the <u>hammer</u> — writer — supplier — leader — speaker or the <u>nail</u> — reader — consumer — follower — audience. The hammer and the nail were designed to build the world together and create good not to destroy. Become the positive hammer and nail of change that you would like to see in the world. Build a better world."

— Brian Michael Good

"The costs to society are much less to feed an open mind with a school meal than to feed a closed mind that no longer has the appetite to believe in the American Dream."

— Brian Michael Good

"The pursuit of the American Dream is alive but not well and may seem obscure and improbable for most of us since is it is harder than ever to achieve with such an abundance of low paying jobs; but the truth is the American Dream has never been easy to attain. Yet, the elusive American Dream is still achievable for anyone with the right attitude, buying behavior, education, savings, knowing the value of hard work, and indomitable will."

— Brian Michael Good

"Let us not mourn the passing of the American Dream just because we have given up hope; many of us are left hoping to win the lottery. Anyone living near or below the poverty line knows very well that the higher cost of services essential for daily survival is a formidable goal for them. Still, many Americans take these blessings for granted."

— Brian Michael Good

"Perception is 98% of reality. Change your perception and you will change your life.

"You don't think that God doesn't know every nuclear launch code in the world!

What are you thinking?

You are making it so easy for God to commence Game Over — Burnt Toast — Nuclear War — Armageddon that we are racing toward is… 100% Guaranteed."

— Brian Michael Good

RESET: You are in: CONTROL Change your perspective: ALT

Forget the past: DELETE

— Brian Michael Good

"Meet your destiny. The contribution of one human's efforts might be the difference between the survival and destruction of humanity."

— Brian Michael Good

Diligence

"Integrity, Honor, Trust, Loyalty, Respect, Reputation. These values should be nurtured as a mother cares for an infant. Without the proper attention, all of these values can be lost from one careless decision."

— Brian Michael Good

"Never look back, never give up, never stop trying, never quit, not even a bit."

— Brian Michael Good

Empathy

"If you suffer from Fear, Anxiety, Anger, or Depression you may be picking up people's feelings and emotions. You might be an <u>Empath</u>."

— Brian Michael Good

"Have kindness, compassion, and empathy towards others and the natural environment."

— Brian Michael Good

"It is nice to be popular but it is popular to be nice."

— Brian Michael Good

"I have a deep sense of compassion and empathy for others; social virtues that I value most in my life."

— Brian Michael Good

Endurance

"Challenges, hardships and obstacles are what life is all about and if you face them with a positive attitude; you will find that it takes half the effort to overcome them. You will find that the sum of your challenges, hardships, and obstacles will define your human spirit and years later as you reflect on your experiences you will realize they have become your strength."

— Brian Michael Good

"A person who navigates life's challenges, hardships and obstacles with stern resolve is able to sail in all winds."

— Brian Michael Good

"You can allow your experiences to destroy you or redefine you. Forget about whom you were; accept who you are, and who you can be.

That is a choice!"

— Brian Michael Good

Environment

"Each individual should strive to live in harmony with the eco-system and the natural environment

— Brian Michael Good

"Climate change as the result of the depletion of our forests, the burning of fossil fuels, large-scale industrial air pollution, environmentally destructive mining methods, irresponsible storage and disposal of contaminants that pollute our air, water and soil should concern all of us. Our planet is essentially being terraformed by mankind's greed. If an alien race was to terraform and warm our planet; we would not allow it. So, why are we allowing mankind's destructive nature to make us sick and kill the planet earth, our only home?"

— Brian Michael Good

"The human race will not survive at the current consumption rate of the top twenty developed countries. By the 2030s, there will be very few third world countries, these countries will have stable developed economies, with large populations that will be vying for the same natural resources and food. I cannot stress this enough. As I said before being spiritual includes protecting the natural environment by practicing the 7Rs?"

— Brian Michael Good

"There's more to well-being than living a spiritual life, it's the state of our planet's future. A spiritual person cares about the environment and sustainability. Being spiritual includes protecting the natural environment by practicing the 7R's…

Reduce your carbon footprint.

Rethink, **Refuse**, **Repurpose**, and **Reuse** items before you discard.

Recycle items that you discard.

Reclaim hazardous waste properly at an eco-collection facility."

— Brian Michael Good

"Individual humans work together with other individual humans but the human race does not work together with nature and the Creator if the human race buys products whose raw materials damage the environment (the Creator's gift) and the wars where humans participate and started/influenced by big business and the wealthy destroy innocent lives."

— Brian Michael Good

"Make a conscious decision to use products for an additional year or two when they contain raw materials that are dangerous (lithium-ion batteries in our cell phones) to transport, hazardous to dispose of back into the environment or may be harmful to the earth in its initial procurement of its raw materials. Purchase manufacturer refurbished products. They are just as good as new items with many of the parts replaced, and sold at far less cost as new product. If you purchase new, be aware that sustainable products do make an environmental impact worldwide, providing economic benefits while protecting the local eco-system that may affect the habitability on Earth, Gaia, and the health of its inhabitants."

— Brian Michael Good

Failure

"Failures are stepping-stones to success and your destiny. Failure allows you to reinvent yourself."

— Brian Michael Good

"You learn more from your mistakes and failures than from any degree of success. Success can only be grasped for a moment before it becomes a distant oasis not to be found again unless you thirst for the knowledge found in the well fed by your mistakes and failures."

— Brian Michael Good

"We are all human, be comfortable with this fact."

— Brian Michael Good

"Never let your attitude be the reason for your failure."

— Brian Michael Good

"Failures are stepping stones to success and your destiny. Failure allows you to reinvent yourself… Instead of looking at your problems as something that is holding you back. View your problems as a solution you haven't found yet."

— Brian Michael Good

"Most of us live our lives in the proactive, reactive, or passive mode. When you are proactive you tend to be positive and prepare for what could happen. When you are reactive you tend to respond when something is about to happen.

A proactive approach can result in a better opportunity for control and fulfillment whereas the reactive mode can result in more stress that can make any problem even more difficult to solve which may lead to failure. A passive life is as if you never lived at all."

— Brian Michael Good

"Sometimes failure or defeat is not an option. You can allow your experiences to destroy you or redefine you. No one can defeat you. You can only defeat yourself."

— Brian Michael Good

"Plan a change. Do something different in your life — move out of your comfort zone. What is most important is the foundation, a step by step outline of your plan that will encourage you to do something different outside your comfort zone. Your plan will likely fail without a step by step outline, the change may not happen if you don't plan or follow through with your plan to venture out of your comfort zone."

— Brian Michael Good

"No success is ever met without a series of failures."

— Brian Michael Good

"I never got my "Big Break" or took full advantage of someone who discovered me and the rest was easy.

So I have decided that I need to take it upon myself to "Break Out Big in 2017."

2017 will be my year… I will have risen from the ashes of defeat…

— Brian Michael Good

Faithfulness

"True faithfulness is often found in the enduring patience of your partner, listening to your long-winded conversations."

— Brian Michael Good

"Trust, faithfulness, and loyalty should define your relationships."

— Brian Michael Good

Family

"Reading a story at bedtime is still a great way for parents to teach their child the lessons necessary for positive social development. If you read stories to your children with morals and virtues until the age of reasoning, they will learn many important life lessons that will help reinforce good behavior as they mature."

— Brian Michael Good

"Children learn more from your actions, and behavior than any lessons obtained from a book or any advice you may give them."

— Brian Michael Good

"Children are not always mature enough to follow advice but often learn from the example of others."

— Brian Michael Good

"Children seldom react well to the harsh tone of your voice, by placing your hand over their mouth, by pulling them by their hands, or by spanking them. Positive reinforcement will help your children to develop a positive self-esteem. Positive reinforcement works far better than any form of discipline that causes excessive fear or anxiety in your child's development."

— Brian Michael Good

"Your children are born with free will. You cannot control their free will without consequences. You are meant to be their guides."

— Brian Michael Good

"Obey your parents, move out and you will find out life could be much harder. You will find that living on the streets and doing whatever it takes to survive will be much harder than living with your parents. Move out only if you might kill yourself or if you are being abused."

— Brian Michael Good

"If you control your body, emotions, and desires, you will be in control of the family finances in your future marriage/relationship."

— Brian Michael Good

"In any good marriage, a woman's voice is equal to man's voice. The same should be true in our open society. Yes, women count as much as men. They count even more than men do, if you consider that women can do what men have considered to be "their domain" of feats, work, sports, business accomplishments, and bear children. You have to admit Women are equal to men."

— Brian Michael Good

"You may choose to be a mother or father someday. However, you will have to earn your acceptance as a good role model and gain respect from your child every day. Acceptance from our children can no longer be taken for granted in any society."

— Brian Michael Good

"Try not to make my mistake (rejection of my daughter); the best thing you can achieve in life is raising a good human by being in their life every day. Children and teenagers need both parents. I wish I had taken some kind of parent training but I guess you have to walk the right path."

— Brian Michael Good

"Most people like to blame someone else and not themselves… In essence they are judging others…

"Take responsibility for any action or reaction you have with your children and others. Once, my daughter jumped on me with such enthusiasm and embrace when I was about to have a bowl of soup that I placed on the wooden arm of the sofa.

I blew the call, when my daughter jumped on me, with all love for her father when she made this innocent, enthusiastic jump of joy. The bowl of soup spilled all over the floor; I said to her, "Why did you make the soup spill?"

"The soup made a mess of the floor and rug. I was the one responsible because I put the soup bowl on the arm of the sofa.

Little did I realize that at nine years old it was the last time she would embrace me with such enthusiasm of her love for me.

Remember, if the soup spills on the floor next time it will be my fault entirely, never again your fault."

— Brian Michael Good

"Nothing of lasting value is given for free; except for the morals, virtues, and lessons taught by our parents."

— Brian Michael Good

"Respect a woman... First impressions are important...

Respect should be consistent by financially supporting and participating with chores and the responsibilities of raising a family."

— Brian Michael Good

"Working is a pleasure... When providing for the ones you love... is your happiness."

— Brian Michael Good

Fear

"You will not to be held captive by fear, anxiety or depression."

— Brian Michael Good

"Fear decreases in exact proportion to your increase in hope."

— Brian Michael Good

"You can't spend your whole life afraid of the rain; you must leave your comfort zone, learn to dance in the rain by accepting the fact that you cannot control everything in life."

— Brian Michael Good

"You are chained by your decision to accept the fear, scars, and pain that you allowed others to bestow on you. It was your acceptance of their mistreatment that stops you from being able to heal from all the attacks. You have the key once you discover that the fear, scars, and pain were self-inflected. Just unlock your chains. A choice."

— Brian Michael Good

"You have only your own perception of reality to fear. If you don't like it… Change it… We all have the power to do something. You have free will."

— Brian Michael Good

"Some of us compromise with their fear, some of us adapt to their fear, some of us are consumed by their fear, some of us are defeated by their fear, and some of us overcome their fear. Confronting fear is an instinctive response for survival. To be held captive by fear in any form is always a choice."

— Brian Michael Good

"Fear is a choice. Feeling paralyzed with fear is not an option. Just be fearless. It might be your only way to save yourself from fear. Fear can consume you and spit you out dead."

— Brian Michael Good

"Fear not. Never look back, never give up, never stop trying, never quit, not even a bit."

— Brian Michael Good

"Life's journey often requires great courage to overcome our greatest fears."

— Brian Michael Good

"Don't be fearful of the future. Own it by allowing yourself to absorb only the positive energy of the people you choose to surround yourself in your new life instead of the negative energy of the old crowd."

— Brian Michael Good

"The evil in your life is the abuse you allow others to bestow on you.
So, if you are a survivor like me and others like me, just be fearless.
It might be your only way to save yourself from fear. Fear can
consume you and spit you out dead."

— Brian Michael Good

"You can't stay in the nest your whole life; you must leave your
comfort zone, spread your wings, and learn to fly on your own."

— Brian Michael Good

Friendship

"Stop feeling sorry for yourself because only you can save yourself. Pick yourself up, go take a walk, meet a new friend or ask someone out on a date. Meet a new friend that will make you laugh."

— Brian Michael Good

"You never know who your friends are. It could be your wife and you better make her your best friend because she knows you like a book and you are well read by her."

— Brian Michael Good

"When you graduate high school or college, you may have made your last friend except if you have the opportunity to make a friend at work or with your partner. But you always have yourself."

— Brian Michael Good

"Develop new friendships; it may be the reason you live."

— Brian Michael Good

"If you want to be respected, try listening to others first. You will make friends and be loved."

— Brian Michael Good

"A person who chooses luxuries as prudently as they should choose their friendships will have a greater opportunity to be rewarded in the afterlife."

— Brian Michael Good

"Try not to create your own loneliness by staying with the old you by not having an awakening. Acceptance is a gift and you get more acceptance than you give. Try to listen first, be more quiet and at peace. You will discover that people will call you, they will invite your friendship, and you will be loved."

— Brian Michael Good

Forgiveness

"When you forgive… You will have made the decision to move forward. Only you can heal yourself. It is a choice."

— Brian Michael Good

"Start a new journey filled with the passion and the love and forgiveness that you deserve."

— Brian Michael Good

"Trust, faithfulness, and loyalty should define your relationships."

— Brian Michael Good

"Forgiveness removes fear. Forgiving others who have hurt you will help you heal. How you view your life will help you to survive."

— Brian Michael Good

"Forgiving is not forgetting; it's actually remembering by not becoming an abuser; yet, using your free will not to hit back with anger or revenge. It's an opportunity for a new beginning, a second chance, a learning experience by not allowing anyone to hurt or abuse you again."

— Brian Michael Good

Free Will

"Free will allows us to paint the canvas of how we choose to live our lives."

— Brian Michael Good

"We are born with free will, a soul, and a ticket to the afterlife. Decide to keep your ticket to the afterlife by never surrendering your soul. Count yourself a survivor."

— Brian Michael Good

"Free will is our greatest gift after life itself, that being said, Free will must be exercised wisely. As much as is humanly possible."

— Brian Michael Good

"Do not attempt to control anyone's free will."

— Brian Michael Good

"We can choose to steer off course or amend it. We have choices. You have free will."

— Brian Michael Good

"If you decide to walk the path of life in complete control of your free will you must resist mind control by adopting a knowledge or faith belief system that is aided with logic and facts."

— Brian Michael Good

"A person whose thoughts are exercised with free will has much more clarity than the thoughts of those who readily accept mind control."

— Brian Michael Good

"Eighty percent of all suicides fail. What, are you crazy? Your free will is taken away. Your life becomes far worse than it is now. Your life is a total mess as a result of your decision."

— Brian Michael Good

"Your children are born with free will. You cannot control their free will without consequences. You are meant to be their guide. If you read your children stories about angels or stories of virtues from a suitable book for children until the age of reasoning, they will learn many important life lessons that will help reinforce good behavior in your children as they mature. Positive reinforcement works far better than any form of discipline that causes excessive fear or anxiety in your child's development."

— Brian Michael Good

"Train yourself to think these thoughts, "I have free will. It is my choice." I suggest that if put a new plan into action and stay with this new attitude about how you might choose to view and live your life; you will positively have more happy moments than ever before in your lifetime."

— Brian Michael Good

"You are born with free will; you can give up or try to live."

— Brian Michael Good

"We all have free will that allows us to move forward by overcoming our self-pity. No one can defeat you. You can only defeat yourself. And that is a choice."

— Brian Michael Good

"Hoping for an entitlement is not what President Franklin Delano Roosevelt meant during his "Four Freedoms Speech" in his State of the Union Address on January 6, 1941: "The freedom of speech, the freedom of worship, the freedom from want, and the freedom from fear." "Freedom from want," means you have the responsibility to provide for your own needs and the free will to pursue the occupation of your choice."

— Brian Michael Good

"Proper training in self-defense can help our children learn self-control of their free will, allowing each of them to develop the self-confidence to walk away from other types of aggression knowing that the best form of self-defense comes from knowing that no one can defeat you. You can only defeat yourself."

— Brian Michael Good

"There are visual stimuli influencing your thoughts as to what happiness should be. A form of mind control. Happiness comes from owning your free will by controlling your thoughts with realistic expectations."

— Brian Michael Good

"Your children are born with free will. You cannot control their free will without consequences. You are meant to be their guides."

— Brian Michael Good

"Find a man/woman/partner that will appreciate everything about you who won't try to change you or control your free will."

— Brian Michael Good

Generosity

"I am fortunate to live in a country where people believe in giving others a second chance."

— Brian Michael Good

"The Creator does not value money but Creator does care where your money came from and what you did with your money as you earned and spent it. It is what you do with your money for people of need."

— Brian Michael Good

"Authority, control, and wealth come with great responsibility. The Creator expects major shareholders, management and business owners to pay honest wages for an honest day's work. Greed does not give you any reward in the afterlife. You have already taken more than your fair share."

— Brian Michael Good

"Luxuries are not a necessity and someday we will realize that the money spent on luxuries could have greatly influenced most of the world's problems."

— Brian Michael Good

"How can the Creator justify retention of wealth when seventeen thousand children a day are dying of hunger? Over four hundred million go hungry on a daily basis, seven hundred and fifty million people do not have access to clean water, 1.2 billion people do not have access to electricity, 2.5 billion people lack adequate sanitation, and billions of people live without affordable housing? "

— Brian Michael Good

Gossip

"News always turns into gossip and gossip always turns into news. Only if you repeat it. It is a choice."

— Brian Michael Good

"The difference between gossip and news heard or seen in social media is getting harder to distinguish between what is true or not true. Best not to repeat what you hear or see even if it is verified. Then ask yourself whether you may be judging that person the same way they may be judged when you share the gossip or news."

— Brian Michael Good

"Rumors, hearsay and gossip are a one-sided story, a distortion of information because every time you gossip something in the story changes. This can cause misunderstandings, which can be a two-way street. When you spread rumors with gossip, it can affect how your peers view you. No one will ever trust you and thus you will not invite true friendships."

— Brian Michael Good

"Avoid gossip, bullying, rumors, hearsay, hazing, harassment, shaming, shunning, and slurs"

— Brian Michael Good

"The truth about gossip is the misinformation that is created can influence a teenager or anyone else' decision to die by suicide. Gossip can kill someone emotionally, mentally, physically and spiritually"

— Brian Michael Good

"If you participate in the gossip, you will be part of the chain of gossip that caused another person to repeat it after you. You may not know that the gossip that you participated in is spreading like fire. You may never know how far your gossip has traveled. If the gossip doesn't start in the first place or if you decide not to participate by refusing to listen to gossip; then the wildfire won't grow rapidly and the firefighters called the peacemakers don't need to called into action to put out the flames"

— Brian Michael Good

"You may not believe you will pay for your gossip. You might not even know that you need to be reflective. Everyone that participates in the gossip is at fault. If you gossip about someone then you may be judged by the Creator. The Creator considers the weak to be his special children even if they are adults. If you gossip over and over again you do not have the Creator in your heart and you just don't get it! You may be surrendering your soul."

— Brian Michael Good

Gratitude

"I spent three months in rehab and the next eight months at a homeless shelter in Cambridge, Massachusetts. That is when I realized that I had not appreciated how much I had before I attempted suicide."

— Brian Michael Good

"Everything we take for granted is a gift; most of us only realize its value upon its loss."

— Brian Michael Good

"Without the help of strangers, my recovery from my cancer and suicide attempt would have been quite difficult."

— Brian Michael Good

"There is no such thing as luck; everything good we experience in our lives is a gift and a blessing."

— Brian Michael Good

"You must find a way to live well even if you did not get the proper guidance from your parents, because you are the one who is responsible for your own life and the decisions you make. It is your choice."

— Brian Michael Good

"There is no such thing as luck, everything we take for granted is a gift and a blessing, and most of us only realize its value upon its loss."

— Brian Michael Good

"Appreciate what the Creator gave you by using what you have been given to the best of your ability."

— Brian Michael Good

Guidance

"What you say does make a difference…

Think of this motto before you react or respond to any situation:

The 4 R's…Readiness, Respect, Right, and Reaction..."

— Brian Michael Good

"Your perception is ninety-eight percent of your reality."

— Brian Michael Good

"There no better gift to another person than the gift of knowledge and understanding derived from wisdom."

— Brian Michael Good

"You are responsible for your own choices, actions, and results."

— Brian Michael Good

"You must find a way to live well even if you don't get the proper guidance from your parents because you are the one who is responsible for your own life and the decisions you make."

— Brian Michael Good

"Pass laws eliminating the compensation that pharmaceuticals pay to doctors and hospitals."

— Brian Michael Good

"No more political action committees PAC's or money from lobbyists. All campaigns should be funded equally using government funds."

— Brian Michael Good

"I propose the formation of the Pacific Treaty Organization – PTO similar in scope to the NATO organization in Europe to offset China's aggression in the South China Sea...Most of the Asian and South Pacific nations that have signed the Trans-Pacific Partnership Nations need to form PTO.

Singapore, Brunei, New Zealand, Australia, Vietnam, Malaysia, Japan are part of the treaty. The Philippines, South Korea, and Indonesia have expressed an interest."

— Brian Michael Good

"Geneva is where the United Nations headquarters should be and hopefully more neutral. The Permanent Five of the United Nations Security Council who have veto power do not represent the present globalization of our world. They represent mostly their own interests and agenda."

— Brian Michael Good

The Permanent Five members include the United States, the U.S.S.R., France, the United Kingdom, and China should not be the only nations on this council. Four of the Permanent Five nations are the World's largest arms exporters. Germany is number five, the United Kingdom is number six and Israel is number seven.

I doubt they want a Peaceful World.

France and the United Kingdom's status should be re-evaluated; they are no longer world powers with sizable populations.

India, a newly formed nation in 1950 after the council was formed should have a seat on the council based on their population and land mass. The nations of my proposed South Pacific Treaty Organization should have a seat on the council.

The European Union, formed in 1951 after the council was formed should have one seat that represents all of them on the council. The EU countries are Austria, Belgium, Bulgaria, Croatia, Republic of Cyprus, Czech Republic, Denmark, Estonia, Finland, France, Germany, Greece, Hungary, Ireland, Italy, Latvia, Lithuania, Luxembourg, Malta, Netherlands, Poland, Portugal, Romania, Slovakia, Slovenia, Spain, and Sweden.

The countries of South America and Africa should each have one seat on the council. Each continent will have one seat and one vote.

There will be now be seven votes not including France, the United Kingdom and the majority rules on all United Nations Security Council votes and no Security Council member is allowed to block any measure like they have in the past."

— Brian Michael Good

"The hungry children of our world need the creation of an international Smart Start Nutrition Program that would provide two nutritious meals, breakfast, a lunch, and a snack to be eaten towards the end of the school day to all pupils in compulsory education regardless of their ability to pay."

Smart Start Nutrition would be the first step in providing an equal educational opportunity that would have a direct correlation to a decrease in the need for international assistance that will diminish the threat of war. Only Sweden, Finland and Estonia provide free school meals to all pupils in compulsory education regardless of their ability to pay."

— Brian Michael Good

"The USA and other nations should return stolen land to indigenous peoples. This might help curtail the suicide rate for Native Americans which are three times the USA national average and possibly help native's pride and hope in other countries."

— Brian Michael Good

"Violent extremism of any faith or ideology that seeks to take the free will, maim or kill others should be dealt with without hesitation and with lethal force if necessary. Terrorists should not have the same human rights that we all should be entitled too."

— Brian Michael Good

"In a more Peaceful World anyone with more than enough money should pay it forward. One might ask…why do some of the super-rich need to retain so much wealth? Until their death, retaining the majority of their wealth will never be acceptable."

— Brian Michael Good

"Authority, control, and wealth come with great responsibility. Major shareholders, management, and business owners to pay honest wages for an honest day's work. Greed does not give you any reward in the afterlife. You have already taken more than your fair share."

— Brian Michael Good

"Have kindness, compassion, and empathy towards others and the natural environment. There's more to well-being than living a more peaceful life, it's the state of our planet's future. A peaceful person cares about the environment and sustainability. Let us show the world how best to live by reducing our ecological footprint and its environmental impact. Being more peaceful includes protecting the natural environment by practicing the 7R's...

• Reduce your carbon footprint.

• Rethink, Refuse, Repurpose, and Reuse items before you discard.

• Recycle items that you discard.

• Reclaim hazardous waste properly at an eco-collection facility. Free.

— Brian Michael Good

"Climate warming will cause food shortages around the word. Proper food storage is the key to extending the expiration date of food allowing you cut food costs by twenty-five percent, giving your family more discretionary income to eat healthier, and helping the environment by avoiding waste."

— Brian Michael Good

"Every place where there is ethnic conflict a 100,000 couples should marry each other. Each person should have a different faith and culture. In five years you'll have so many babies that chances are there will be less conflict."

— Brian Michael Good

"No more human trafficking or child labor. No more Czars. No more blood money. Cut the crime rate."

— Brian Michael Good

"A closed mind is like a parachute malfunction, a mind like a parachute only works if it is fully open."

— Brian Michael Good

"A human being is not what you are but who you can become if you choose to awaken to a greater reality. Most of us never attempt to grasp this."

— Brian Michael Good

"It is part of our human nature to question what we know and what we don't know."

— Brian Michael Good

"Each individual should focus on their own personal spiritual life; be aware that you may be surrendering your soul in your judgment or treatment of others."

— Brian Michael Good

"It may take you a lifetime to figure which direction you are headed but it might because when you were young you were never given a track to run on."

— Brian Michael Good

"Ninety percent of us exist, ten percent of us live. Choose to live well. Choose to live life to the fullest. Most of all, we should all do our Best to Live."

— Brian Michael Good

"In any good marriage, a woman's voice is equal to man's voice. The same should be true in our open society. Yes, women count as much as men. They count even more than men do, if you consider that women can do what men have considered to be "their domain" of feats, work, sports, business accomplishments, and bearing children. You have to admit Women are equal to men."

— Brian Michael Good

"We should not commercially hunt, allow testing, or separate any mammal from their family or social unit. Many mammals have similar emotional characteristics as humans. Who is to say they do not have souls, when many people believe that, their cat or dog will go to heaven. Just because we believe that human beings are the highest part of Creator's (God's) creation, does not make it so.

We have yet to explore the universe where there are estimated to be billions of Earth like planets. We might discover truths that would be inconceivable within our present day reality. Just because we have always hunted does not make it right to instill fear in the mammal we hunt.

Except for providing food for your family, thou shall not kill might pertain to many mammals of the animal kingdom."

— Brian Michael Good

"We must stop the present day slow genocide of Native Americans, the Aborigines of all nations, and their culture. Why are we still doing this? The USA views themselves as a Christian Nation… We need to be Spiritual Nations.

There is little difference from what the settlers and the USA government (a Christian nation) did to the Native Americans and what the Catholic Church did during the Roman Catholic Inquisition. The Catholic Church had a history of collecting property and wealth from the dead after killing and torturing millions of Christians and

Jews during the hundreds of years of the Roman Catholic Inquisition.

Over 500 treaties made with American Indian tribes were broken when it was to the United States government's advantage. The USA government helps its citizens in their recovery from national disasters. Yet, the present day genocide continues when Teen Suicide on American Indian reservations is almost three times the national rate, radiation from a nuclear dump threatens the Navajo/Hopi water supply, poor nutrition for many Native Americans has persisted for decades, and Apache sacred land was recently given to a copper company when a provision was approved by Congress."

— Brian Michael Good

"It is a War on Drugs!

God allows you to protect your society and its people.

War on Drugs should include stopping people from "abusing legal drugs.

Be forewarned... Do not kill an innocent person. Only military and law enforcement can protect the public not private citizens.

God allows self-defense. I agree with killing people who are part of the drug culture. I do not agree with untrained/unauthorized private citizens being involved.

Afghanistan, Burma (Myanmar), Mexico, Colombia, Peru, Bolivia, China, and the Bahamas are the leading countries who manufacture and grow illegal drugs.

Any person who to part of the illegal drug business: manufacturing farming process... owners, investors, shareholders, stock brokers, manufacturing personnel, shipment, actions or selling of a drugs that maims, kills, or instills fear towards an innocent person either directly or indirectly should be dealt with without hesitation and with lethal force if necessary.

Those involved with the drug culture should not have the same human rights that we all should be entitled too."

Their action results in the collateral damage of drug-related theft, and instills fear, the sexual exploitation and killing of God's children; as a result they shall receive God's judgement and vengeance."

— Brian Michael Good

"The human race Sucks... Humans take land, wealth, ruin lives, enslave, use mind control, kill humans, rape, pillage for greed and power like a virus.

Thus, the human race is a virus that cannot be allowed to infect the universe.

The human race must Change or be Quarantine - Contained - Isolated in your solar system or Destroyed - Eradicated at any cost."

— Brian Michael Good

Happiness

"You are in the center of your happiness when you pursue your passion."

— Brian Michael Good

"Be a lifeline for someone who needs your support. We will be undefeated in our pursuit of happiness. Be part of a Life Squad and find someone who needs a friend to lean on."

— Brian Michael Good

"How you manage your expectations is the secret to happiness and finding peace in your life."

— Brian Michael Good

"Peace and happiness are renewed for those who seek it."

— Brian Michael Good

"Accepting yourself the way you are is the secret to happiness and finding peace in your life."

— Brian Michael Good

"For many of us, it takes decades to realize that happiness comes from within us."

— Brian Michael Good

"Happiness is how our conscious thoughts react in harmony with the external sources and stimuli in our world."

— Brian Michael Good

"I realized that money gave me temporary happiness. As I matured to an adult, I began not to value money when my inability to sustain a consistent income became my new, but hopefully not permanent, reality."

— Brian Michael Good

"Now you know that life's happiness is all about your decision on how you react. It is never too late to take this road with thorns called life to where you want to be at. We are all human, be comfortable with this fact."

— Brian Michael Good

"Break the cycle. Create your own world of good and happiness."

— Brian Michael Good

"Choose to begin to change one day at a time, tiny steps where you position yourself in a steady motion of happiness and tranquility instead of allowing yourself to be hashed around beyond your control."

— Brian Michael Good

"There are visual stimuli influencing your thoughts as to what happiness should be. A form of mind control. Happiness comes from owning your free will by controlling your thoughts with realistic expectations."

— Brian Michael Good

"Elements Found in Happiness — Life, Free will, "Your soul – "your very essence", Dominion over other species, Sustenance, Shelter, Hope, Gratification, Love, Friendship, Creativity, Passion, and Destiny."

— Brian Michael Good

"The happiest moments that unite us as humans are when we enjoy music, dance, friends, family, and the birth of a child."

— Brian Michael Good

"Listening to others is a key to our survival. Laughter is very important to our well-being. You feel healthier and happier?"

— Brian Michael Good

"Being in the company of friends and family or being a couple with someone is a temporary illusion. We are born alone, we are alone with our own thoughts, and we go to the afterlife alone.

Be happy with your own company... Me, Myself, and I.

It is the most permanent form of happiness."

— Brian Michael Good

"A truly happy person is one who can control their stress by deciding to get enough sleep, meditate, exercise, proper diet, nature/outdoor breaks, and less dependence on cell phone and social media."

— Brian Michael Good

"Just do the very best you can do. Create a fresh attitude by changing your perspective; the way you think will go a long way in making you happy. Acceptance is the key. To forgive is to let GO.

You must RESET:

You are in: CONTROL
Change your perspective: ALT
Forget the past: DELETE."

— Brian Michael Good

Hatred

"We are all exposed to the harsh realities of life. There is always going to be someone or a group of people who don't like you."

— Brian Michael Good

"Forgiving is not forgetting; it's actually remembering by not becoming an abuser; by using your free will not to hit back with anger, hatred, or revenge. It's an opportunity for a new beginning, a second chance, a learning experience by not allowing anyone to hurt or abuse you again."

— Brian Michael Good

Healing

\---------------------------------

"I have come to realize that without the engine; the body, getting a tune-up; the driver, the mind, cannot get where it wants to go in life very well. A healthy mind begins with a healthy body and vice versa."

— Brian Michael Good

\---------------------------------

"Sticks and stones may break your bones but you will decide if the words and names will ever hurt you. No one can defeat you. You can only defeat yourself. That is a choice."

— Brian Michael Good

\---------------------------------

"No one can defeat you. You can only defeat yourself. No one can truly save you. You must save yourself."

— Brian Michael Good

\---------------------------------

"Just let it GO and with fun, love, friendships, and laughter... You can choose to heal."

— Brian Michael Good

\---------------------------------

Health

"I do not drink liquor or beer on a regular basis and I no longer smoke cigarettes; the benefits go beyond my physical heath for my refrigerator and shelves and my life have an abundance of food that is now affordable."

— Brian Michael Good

"Some of us will experience some form of mental illness in their lifetime… I rather have depression that can be treated with a pill and my free will to conquer it; than have a physical illness that results in my demise because no matter what I did I could not conquer it."

— Brian Michael Good

"Think about a car not having ample petro/gas to start the engine, as the body not getting the proper nutrition, preventing the driver from arriving at their desired destination.

An engaged mind likewise cannot develop the knowledge base on life skills that will be needed to achieve upward mobility."

— Brian Michael Good

"I have come to realize that without the engine; the body, getting a tune-up; the driver, the mind, cannot get where it wants to go in life very well. A healthy mind begins with a healthy body and vice versa."

— Brian Michael Good

"A person who is a little bit insane may be saner than someone who is completely sane. A little bit of insanity gives a person a better perspective on what the difference is between perception and reality."

— Brian Michael Good

"The clock's ticking… The longer you wait to change your life the harder it becomes to implement change. Sixty years old is mid-life if you consider that a healthy person with modern medical care might live to one hundred twenty. So what are you waiting for?"

— Brian Michael Good

"Everyone deserves a "Me" day without any guilt or regret... Relax and enjoy a day off."

— Brian Michael Good

"Listening to others is a key to our survival. Laughter is very important to our well-being. You feel healthier and happier?"

— Brian Michael Good

Honor

"Originality is as RARE as finding an honest person. So many people on social media never give the author credit for use of their quote."

— Brian Michael Good

"Do not steal anything in any way."

— Brian Michael Good

"Integrity and honor should be part of every fabric of your beliefs."

— Brian Michael Good

"There is no honor in any killing. No family has the right to an "honor killing" when they kill a female relative."

— Brian Michael Good

"Honesty is very rare in our world and it is hard to find it in social media. Maybe we should favorite, retweet, like or add a quote to our social media a quote on social media only when the author is given proper credit."

— Brian Michael Good

"Just because it may be easy to go to peer-to-peer network and pirate or download a movie, music, or program free of charge does not mean you are not stealing it. Just because it is easy to share or copy your friend's music does not mean you are not stealing it. You have free will. Everything is a choice."

— Brian Michael Good

Hope

"Hope should never be extinguished; hope like the flame of a torch should be transferred to another torch before it flickers out allowing your hope to burn brightly again."

— Brian Michael Good

"You may not fully recover but you can adapt. The next battle is often won by finding a new source of hope that will push you forward."

— Brian Michael Good

"Acceptance of your failure is not an excuse to give up on any situation but to temporary accept defeat in order to retreat when the battle is lost to live to fight the battle another day with a new plan of action that gives you hope that victory is still attainable. You may not fully recover but you can adapt. The next battle is often won by finding a new source of hope that will push you forward."

— Brian Michael Good

"A dream not yet realized offers far more benefits than the reality one faces when they give up hope."

— Brian Michael Good

"To travel with hope is more important than arriving at your destination."

— Brian Michael Good

"Never give up hope; for without hope; food, water, faith or beliefs will not be enough to nourish your body, mind and soul."

— Brian Michael Good

Humility

"It is difficult to be humble when you are recognized for your achievements. It is better to keep your achievements to yourself by staying under the radar and remain humble."

— Brian Michael Good

"There is more beauty in someone who is humble than someone who sees themselves as perfect."

— Brian Michael Good

"If you become successful, some may be jealous. The more humble and private you are; the less jealous they will be; and the more true friendships you will have..."

— Brian Michael Good

Inspiration

"You cannot rush inspiration, for inspiration comes from the body, mind, soul, and the cosmos."

— Brian Michael Good

"I have great resolve. I use what you did to me (steal and rejection) to tear me down to motivate and inspire myself.

No one can defeat you. You can only defeat yourself. No one can save you. You must save yourself."

— Brian Michael Good

"Each person's destiny is unique, some are destined to be great; some are destined to inspire greatness and change in others.

We can be only be great for a stitch in time; we shine only for a moment in God's favor and greatness; and then we are forgotten. I rather be a positive influence on others, it is the only great way to become immortal, for inspiration never truly dies for it instills hope"

— Brian Michael Good

"Inspiration and hope should never be extinguished; hope is like the flame of a torch, each generation needs inspiration that is transferred to another torch before the flame flickers out, allowing hope to burn brightly again."

BRIAN MICHAEL GOOD

— Brian Michael Good

Jealousy

"Why would you be jealous when you have free will to strive for anything you want?"

— Brian Michael Good

"If you become successful, some may be jealous. The more humble and private you are; the less jealous they will be; and the more true friendships you will have…"

— Brian Michael Good

Judgement

"Avoid judgment of ethnic, racial, sexual orientation, gender identity, and religious differences in society."

— Brian Michael Good

"No one is all good nor is one person all bad."

— Brian Michael Good

"The color of my skin at birth was white. It is several layers deep. If I shine an ultraviolet lamp on my skin which emits pure UV (no visible light), it shows that my skin is actually multicolored. I chose to wear my skin multicolored."

— Brian Michael Good

"At some point in your life, you may wonder if your soul is hanging by a thread. This thread is the conduit in which your belief system flows defining your human spirit and binding to the fabric of your soul. Religious, Philosophical, and Ideological fibers are spun into a single strand giving strength to your beliefs. It is this thread's strength that allows you to be broad-minded and even-handed. Be aware that you may be surrendering your soul in your judgment or treatment of others."

— Brian Michael Good

"We may be judged on what we could have done when you had a moral obligation to help someone in need. You have free will. It is your choice."

— Brian Michael Good

"Do not judge your lot in life and do not over judge yourself. Do not feel sorry for yourself. Stop whining. Do not self-pity. Life can always be worse than it is. Nothing is the end of the world. There is always a way to fix it."

— Brian Michael Good

"Millions of years ago the entire human species might have been hermaphrodites, having both testicular and ovarian tissue which is present in one percent of all mammals including humans. If humans are still born with both reproductive tissues then this might explain that our species might have been biologically gay or transgender from the very beginning.

Using knowledge, reason, and logic may help to understand what we do not understand. We may have always been gay or transgender as a species but only in the past 6,000 years, religious dogma has taught us it was taboo to be homosexual. Be careful who you judge, only We-she-me-he – God – The Creator – Universe knows the truth."

— Brian Michael Good

"Decide to keep your ticket to the afterlife by never surrendering your soul, for God's judgment is inescapable."

— Brian Michael Good

"Most people like to blame someone else and not themselves… In essence they are judging others…

"Take responsibility for any action or reaction you have with your children and others. Once, my daughter jumped on me with such enthusiasm and embrace when I was about to have a bowl of soup that I placed on the wooden arm of the sofa.

I blew the call, when my daughter jumped on me, with all love for her father when she made this innocent, enthusiastic jump of joy. The bowl of soup spilled all over the floor; I said to her, "Why did you make the soup spill?"

"The soup made a mess of the floor and rug. I was the one responsible because I put the soup bowl on the arm of the sofa.

Little did I realize that at nine years old it was the last time she would embrace me with such enthusiasm of her love for me.

Remember, if the soup spills on the floor next time it will be my fault entirely, never again your fault."

— Brian Michael Good

Kindness

"Have kindness, compassion, and empathy towards others and the natural environment."

— Brian Michael Good

"Help someone in need with kindness including yourself."

— Brian Michael Good

"When you do an act of kindness to others, you are really doing a kindness to yourself; for during the act of kindness you are not thinking of your own problems and will receive back the gratitude even if it is just a smile."

— Brian Michael Good

"Peace sprouts only from the love and kindness showed towards another human or creature. Peace is renewed from the love and kindness showed to others."

— Brian Michael Good

Knowledge

"There no better gift to another person than the gift of knowledge and understanding derived from wisdom."

— Brian Michael Good

"Humans have become more logical, facts build our knowledge and belief system. A logical person gathers facts and does not rely on faith alone."

— Brian Michael Good

"We are gravitating towards building a knowledge belief system that is constructed mainly on materials based on facts.

— Brian Michael Good

"Survival often requires not only knowledge and wisdom but the willingness to adapt to new challenges."

— Brian Michael Good

"There is enough wealth in our world to teach and share knowledge so each town or village can provide their own food, shelter, clothing and other commodities and services that are essential for survival."

— Brian Michael Good

"If you decide to walk the path of life in complete control of your free will you must resist mind control by adopting a knowledge or faith belief system that is aided with logic and facts."

— Brian Michael Good

"Think about a car not having ample petro/gas to start the engine, as the body not getting the proper nutrition, preventing the driver from arriving at their desired destination.

An engaged mind likewise cannot develop the knowledge base on life skills that will be needed to achieve upward mobility."

— Brian Michael Good

"You learn more from your mistakes and failures than from any degree of success. Success can only be grasped for a moment before it becomes a distant oasis not to be found again unless you thirst for the knowledge found in the well fed by your mistakes and failures."

— Brian Michael Good

Loyalty

"Trust, faithfulness, and loyalty should define your relationships."

— Brian Michael Good

"Integrity, Honor, Trust, Loyalty, Respect, Reputation. These values should be nurtured as a mother cares for an infant. Without the proper attention, all of these values can be lost from one careless decision."

— Brian Michael Good

Love

"Lovers have ripped out my heart... Emptiness remains, yet I still bleed...

I think of how lovers have taken my bleeding heart from me. What's left of the space where my heart was once safe... it still bleeds. It is my hope that the empty space where my heart and romantic love once were will never bleed again.

I have been through lots of heartaches... My heart has been broken on numerous occasions, each time it needs time to heal... Often, just like a Bleeding Hearts Plant bleeds as it matures, I do not have a choice as I witness the heartache as the result of men's rejection and the abandonment of their growing families...

Many of us grew up with a childhood where love flourished in my heart which was provided/supported by parents, grandparents, friends, and extended family who nurtured a consistent family atmosphere that created a warm, safe, loving and peaceful life.

The love that was once long by a suitor to capture my heart is now forgotten by them; yet it still lingers in my thoughts. This heart is no longer living in the past for I can feel my heart warm as I look quietly and gaze as my soulmate walks in and out of my life. It is my thoughts of my heart's rejection of love that stops me from the romantic happiness I truly seek.

Sadly, the seeds of love that was once vital for nourishment of my growing heart are no longer seeded for it is my choice to open my heart again in order for the seeds of love to be planted again.

The abuse is often forgiven as time heals; often we decide to keep our heart closed for it will not open naturally.

When you finally realized that your heart is now healthy, it will be your decision to move forward. A warmed heart sprouts from seeds of love only from a desired future with another.

It is our own free will choice to love again…

— Brian Michael Good

"I love you with all the love I have gathered in my lifetime."

— Brian Michael Good

"I have no doubt there is a Creator and that the Creator loves and cares about all of us. When we were given the gift of free will, our greatest gift after life itself, we were expected to solve our own problems. When you look to the Creator for guidance, do it knowing that it is your responsibility to find a solution."

— Brian Michael Good

"If you want to control your lover then do not even think of controlling them. When you do not try to control your partner in a relationship, then you are in control and your partner will always be at your side as your best friend. You will receive far more love and respect than a person who wants control in a relationship."

— Brian Michael Good

"Find a man/woman/partner that will appreciate everything about you who won't try to change you or control your free will."

— Brian Michael Good

"I know the tide that has not come to shore in over several years will greet me like a tidal wave of open embrace."

— Brian Michael Good

"You should be wise who you love and invest your emotions. If you love your soulmate you will seldom get hurt, if at all."

— Brian Michael Good

"Be single. You won't meet your soulmate if you are dating someone. A true soulmate would be wary of any relationship lasting with you if they took you away from another.

They would never fully trust you in a relationship. You would have already shown you are not loyal to the one you are with when you met."

— Brian Michael Good

"Life can be so fragile, sometimes love is what's needed the most."

— Brian Michael Good

"Peace sprouts only from the love and kindness showed towards another human or creature. Peace is renewed from the love and kindness showed to others."

— Brian Michael Good

"Meet your soulmate and there is no need to play the game because both people who are each other's soulmate know the rules and appreciate each other's value enough not to break the rules.

When you meet your soulmate. Take it slow...

Build a foundation first that allows the roots of love to sprout."

— Brian Michael Good

"True faithfulness is often found in the enduring patience of your partner, listening to your long-winded conversations."

— Brian Michael Good

"You know you are pass the honeymoon stage and in the relationship stage when your partner asks you to stop talking.

I love you honey... I'll zip it!"

— Brian Michael Good

Passion

"Every day starts fresh when you have a good night sleep, a passion to pursue and a positive attitude. A choice."

— Brian Michael Good

"Every endeavor in life is not about the odds of success but about your belief, your passion, and your indomitable will."

— Brian Michael Good

"You need to take the necessary steps to put your life on the right course to develop your passion."

— Brian Michael Good

"You are in the center of your happiness when you pursue your passion."

— Brian Michael Good

"Meeting your destiny doesn't happen without a plan, a plan doesn't happen without a purpose, a purpose doesn't happen without finding your passion, a passion isn't discovered without the pursuit of activities that you enjoy."

— Brian Michael Good

"Find a purpose for your life and you will do extraordinary things.

You are in center of your happiness when you pursue your passion.

When you pursue your passion, you are the master of your environment.

"When you are the master of your environment you often meet your destiny."

— Brian Michael Good

Peace

"The best fight won is the fight not fought."

— Brian Michael Good

"Part of the foundation for creating a Peaceful World is to stop the killing of mammals or species that prove proportionately to possess a high level of intelligence and emotions similar to humans. We may not be the only species with souls."

— Brian Michael Good

"If you decide to be the change in the world, and walk the path of life in peace; you must have complete control of your free will, and resist mind control by adopting a knowledge or faith belief system that is aided with logic and facts."

— Brian Michael Good

"What does stand your ground mean to me? A peaceful person...

It means to love myself enough that if you try to tear me down by saying something disrespectful to me.

I will stand up for myself and defend the self-respect that I have for myself. Not in a physical action but I will verbally defend the person I know better than you and have lived with my entire life... Me."

— Brian Michael Good

"Peace sprouts only from the love and kindness showed towards another human or creature. Peace is renewed for those who seek.

When you meet another person or when two or more are gathered you will have the opportunity to create the gift of acceptance, the epitome of what humanity should be!

The higher you raise yourself in the better treatment of others, the better view you will have of the future."

— Brian Michael Good

"We need more peace in the world if the human race is to survive. I need seven billion humans to join in our effort to create a more Peaceful World. If you are about to get in a confrontation, fight, or argument, just say these words; I am Peace. We are Peace...

The I am Peace... We are Peace... pledge does not take away your right to stand your ground or your right to self-defense "What you say and think and how you react does make a difference.

Think of this motto before you react or respond to any situation:

The 4 R's...Readiness, Respect, Right, and Reaction...

Take to heart and own these words as a pledge of honor; say these words first; I am Peace... We are Peace...

That is why we are trying to make a difference. One person at a time, deciding to talk the talk...and walk the walk... each person leading by example can make a difference.

It's all about what you are willing to do out of your own free will. We need to be united in order to create a more Peaceful World on the planet Earth. The right formula that works as a step towards World Peace.

We are all Spirits in a human body; no one does it alone, as one spirit; one united movement, evil can't defeat us.

It all starts with the 4 R's... Readiness, Respect, Right, Reaction; when you greet a person, begin the conversation with these words...

"I am Peace... We are Peace...

Join the "I am Peace... We are Peace...Movement and Pledge...

Take the Pledge. What number will you be?

I am Peace... We are Peace.

— Brian Michael Good

All wars must be fought on the battlefield... If the bomb or bullet is not made then the innocent are not maimed or killed...

Any person who to part of the weaponization process...owners, investors, shareholders, stock brokers, manufacturing personnel, shipment, deployment or firing of a weapon that maims or kills an innocent shall receive God's judgement and vengeance.

— Brian Michael Good

Six percent of the world's population lives in the Middle East, Turkey, Afghanistan Pakistan... Yet, ninety percent of the war and conflict is fought in this area on Earth.

Be forewarned God has decided if you do not start getting along, the world will be better off without this real estate...

— Brian Michael Good

"I am a feminist in the exact definition of the word, I believe in social, political, and all rights to be equal to both women and men. I believe in the equalism movement for all humans, absence of required roles, labels, or behaviors that gender may require. That being said, we need more emphasis that men and women are equal and it should not be a battle of the sexes. Equalism is not a gender issue concerning men or women; it is about treating every human with respect and equality.

The only path to world peace is through women's equality to men. The only way women will be considered equal to men is when the world realizes that women are better than men. Only then will mankind accept that women are their equal. When women are equal to men, women will run the world like they run their families. Do you even think women would allow what's happening in the Middle East, the Ukraine or allow nuclear warheads to be in existence on our planet? Women would not allow the threat of one person having access to the button that would cause Game Over/Armageddon and kill their children or grandchildren.

There is no such thing as limited nuclear war. If one nuclear bomb is successful, then all of them will be eventually launched. Free will comes with a price.... God will not save you. The human race (women) must save themsclves."

"What are you waiting for? The clock's ticking...

Oh... It's a nuclear clock."

— Brian Michael Good

Present

"Acceptance – Let go of the past to get ahead in the present."

— Brian Michael Good

"You can effect change in the present. In the Now!"

— Brian Michael Good

"Live life in the present, in the now and it will happen."

— Brian Michael Good

"All we can really do or control is living in the moment."

— Brian Michael Good

"Dwelling on negatives affects our rhythm and holds us back from the present."

— Brian Michael Good

"Live in the present, where it is the best place to live."

— Brian Michael Good

"Tomorrow becomes Today when Today becomes Tomorrow."

— Brian Michael Good

"You can change the future only by implementing change in the present."

— Brian Michael Good

"If you can feel pain living in the past, forgiving others will help you move into the present."

— Brian Michael Good

"The wisdom in our future is discovered in the present. You cannot go forward unless you let go of the past."

— Brian Michael Good

"Yes, you can replace old memories with new ones and start over in the present. I find that the best place to live is in the now."

— Brian Michael Good

"Acceptance helps you to skip forward and live in the present."

— Brian Michael Good

"What you choose today, you live with tomorrow."

— Brian Michael Good

"Living in the present and being a survivor will be always how I stay in the eye of my hurricane; safe from the storm around me."

— Brian Michael Good

"It has been said that in a lifetime we live many lives. If you don't like your life begin your next life within your present life by implementing change in the present."

— Brian Michael Good

"The present, this moment is all we truly own and are guaranteed. Why not enjoy it."

— Brian Michael Good

Problems

"Do not dwell on problems in which you cannot effect any change."

— Brian Michael Good

"If you have a problem then do everything you can to correct or rectify this problem. You can't change the negatives of the past. Dwelling on negatives affects our rhythm and holds us back in the present. The future may be viewed and anticipated but it is not laid out precisely like a blueprint. You can effect change in the present. We have free will to choose to steer off course or amend it. We have choices."

— Brian Michael Good

"Mind over matter. If it matters; you will put your mind to it. The mind is capable of solving any problem that matters."

— Brian Michael Good

"Many times what is going to happen is just a reaction to what just happened. Break the chain reaction cycles by finding the source of the problem."

— Brian Michael Good

"There is always a reason why things happen. Find the source of the
problem and you will only find the peace that allows you to
go forward by putting the problem behind you."

— Brian Michael Good

Reputation

"We are defined by the decisions we make and the actions we take. Before you respond to any situation, put your brain into gear before you put your mouth or any reaction into motion."

— Brian Michael Good

"What you say does make a difference…

Think of this motto before you react or respond to any situation:

The 4 R's…Readiness, Respect, Right, and Reaction..."

— Brian Michael Good

"Your values have much to do with accomplishing your goals and fulfilling your potential."

— Brian Michael Good

"Integrity, Honor, Trust, Loyalty, Respect, Reputation. These values should be nurtured as a mother cares for an infant. Without the proper attention, all of these values can be lost from one careless decision."

— Brian Michael Good

Respect

"What you say does make a difference...

Think of this motto before you react or respond to any situation:

The 4 R's...Readiness, Respect, Right, and Reaction..."

— Brian Michael Good

"Often respect is like seeing your reflection while looking at the surface of still water."

— Brian Michael Good

"Respect, like your reflection, must be projected first (good manners) in order to see the same reflection of respect returned."

— Brian Michael Good

"Women do eighty percent of the buying and handle the family finances in many households. Yet, the most widely used US dollar bill, the twenty dollar bill is not good enough, nor does the ten dollar bill show enough "Respect" to the women of the United States of America."

— Brian Michael Good

"Respect a woman... First impressions are important...

Respect should be consistent by financially supporting and participating with chores and the responsibilities of raising a family."

— Brian Michael Good

Revenge

"Don't trouble, trouble, or trouble will trouble you."

— Brian Michael Good

"Forgiving is not forgetting; it's actually remembering by not becoming an abuser; yet, using your free will not to hit back with anger or revenge. It's an opportunity for a new beginning, a second chance, a learning experience by not allowing anyone to hurt or abuse you again."

— Brian Michael Good

Scars

"I used to blame others for every hurt and the scars, from the years of abuse (emotionally, physically, and mentally) during my childhood and teenage years, but now, having forgiven them (my abusers) for everything I realize the abuse was self-inflicted. It was my acceptance of their mistreatment. I blame myself for not being able to heal from the hurt and the scars."

— Brian Michael Good

"You cannot go forward unless you let go of the past/scar."

— Brian Michael Good

"You are chained by your decision to accept the fear, scars, and pain that you allowed others to bestow on you. It was your acceptance of their mistreatment that stops you from being able to heal from all the attacks. You have the key once you discover that the fear, scars, and pain were self-inflected. Just unlock your chains. A choice."

— Brian Michael Good

"The thorn in your arm that could have been self-inflicted by you will do you no harm if you know the right facts. That every road has its own thorn that can hold you back from the way you react. That it has always been your decision to accept the hurt and the scars that stops you from not being able to heal from all the attacks. Now that you know that how you react is what makes this to be a fact; it's never too late to take this road with thorns called life to where you want to be at."

— Brian Michael Good

"A scar often reminds us of the past. Sometimes a scar is an invisible wound that was not mended and never healed. When you accept that people do not scar or give you pain; you'll realize that your open wound was self-inflicted. It is your acceptance of their mistreatment that stops the open wound from being healed that prevents you from moving past the hurt that only you view as a scar no matter how fresh or old the wound."

— Brian Michael Good

Soul *"your very essence"*

"The souls of any vessel are the sailors who navigate the ship."

— Brian Michael Good

"At some point in your life, you may wonder if your soul is hanging by a thread. This thread is the conduit in which your belief system flows defining your human spirit and binding to the fabric of your soul. Religious, Philosophical, and Ideological fibers are spun into a single strand giving strength to your beliefs. It is this thread's strength that allows you to be broad-minded and even-handed. Be aware that you may be surrendering your soul in your judgment or treatment of others."

— Brian Michael Good

"Each individual should focus on their own personal spiritual life, aware that they may be surrendering their soul in the judgment or treatment of others."

— Brian Michael Good

"If you are prepared to enter the afterlife, the day you die should be a bigger celebration than the day you are born."

— Brian Michael Good

"We should not commercially hunt, allow testing, or separate any mammal from their family or social unit. Many mammals have similar emotional characteristics as humans. Who is to say they do not have souls, when many people believe that, their cat or dog will go to heaven. Just because we believe that human beings are the highest part of Creator's (God's) creation, does not make it so.

We have yet to explore the universe where there are estimated to be billions of Earth like planets. We might discover truths that would be inconceivable within our present day reality. Just because we have always hunted does not make it right to instill fear in the mammal we hunt.

Except for providing food for your family, thou shall not kill might pertain to many mammals of the animal kingdom."

— Brian Michael Good

"Beauty on this earthly plane is often short lived... A beautiful heart and soul will last an eternity."

— Brian Michael Good

"Decide to keep your ticket to the afterlife by never surrendering your soul, for God's judgment is inescapable."

— Brian Michael Good

Strength

"Challenges, hardships and obstacles are what life is all about and if you face them with a positive attitude; you will find that it takes half the effort to overcome them. You will find that the sum of your challenges, hardships, and obstacles will define your human spirit and years later as you reflect on your experiences you will realize they have become your strength."

— Brian Michael Good

"Today, I will try to stay in the eye of my hurricane where I am safe from the storm around me. I will try to deal with my hurricanes and struggles in life with no blame or excuses.

My hurricanes keep coming. I gain strength with each pearl of wisdom that washes ashore."

— Brian Michael Good

"Challenges, hardships and obstacles are what life is all about and if you face them with a positive attitude; you will find that it takes half the effort to overcome them. You will find that the sum of your challenges, hardships, and obstacles will define your human spirit and years later as you reflect on your experiences you will realize they have become your strength."

— Brian Michael Good

Stress

"Most of us live our lives in the proactive, reactive, or passive mode. When you are proactive you tend to be positive and prepare for what could happen. When you are reactive you tend to respond when something is about to happen.

A proactive approach can result in a better opportunity for control and fulfillment whereas the reactive mode can result in more stress that can make any problem even more difficult to solve which may lead to failure. A passive life is as if you never lived at all."

— Brian Michael Good

"A truly happy person is one who can control their stress by deciding to get enough sleep, meditate, exercise, proper diet, nature/outdoor breaks, and less dependence on cell phone and social media."

— Brian Michael Good

Success

"Every endeavor in life is not about the odds of success but about your belief, your passion, and your indomitable will."

— Brian Michael Good

"Before you can be successful you must have the right perspective and mindset. Seize the day and Recharge your life."

— Brian Michael Good

"A positive attitude influences our behavior and dictates a successful approach."

— Brian Michael Good

"No one can defeat you. You can only defeat yourself. That is a choice."

— Brian Michael Good

"No success is ever met without a series of failures."

— Brian Michael Good

"No human is an island if they want to successful."

BRIAN MICHAEL GOOD

— Brian Michael Good

Tolerance

"Have tolerance and respect towards others and their culture."

— Brian Michael Good

"A person should weigh all twelve of the universal values to live by equally, following one value and not another is as if you follow none of them. The true lesson gained from having good values comes from valuing the rights of others, not just your own."

— Brian Michael Good

"The best fight won is the fight not fought."

— Brian Michael Good

Trust

"Trust and loyalty should define your relationships."

— Brian Michael Good

"Integrity, Honor, Trust, Loyalty, Respect, Reputation. These values should be nurtured as a mother cares for an infant. Without the proper attention, all of these values can be lost from one careless decision."

— Brian Michael Good

"Mind control decays your ability to pursue and discover the truth. Mind control can use fear to control you. Do not let them control your free will with fear. Remove mind control and you will remove fear. Hit the reset button in your brain and live your life with less fear. Follow the truth but follow no one blindly."

— Brian Michael Good

"Be careful of anyone that states everything in a particular book or religion is one hundred percent the truth. There are over four thousand religions in our world and over thirty-four thousand Christian denominations. Only Weshemehe knows all the truth. Respect everyone's free will to search for the truth. Own your human gift of free will by exercising it; read, discover, assimilate, and question anything you want."

— Brian Michael Good

"I will not belong to a place of worship that says I have to believe one hundred percent in their dogma or their unique religious perspective. I refuse to give up my free will to pursue what I believe to be the truth."

— Brian Michael Good

Truth

"Follow the truth but follow no one blindly."

— Brian Michael Good

"No one should resolutely affect your pursuit of the truth."

— Brian Michael Good

"History and religion are often written with a controlled message, a form of mind control."

— Brian Michael Good

"The abuse is often forgiven as time heals, it should never be forgotten; otherwise we will not learn the truth from the past for whatever we chose to forget will be repeated."

— Brian Michael Good

"You will decipher the truth about how to find happiness and meet your destiny. If you haven't developed a passion, concept, or goal for your life and an action plan on the best way to achieve it, you will never know whether you could have made it to a place you once thought was impossible."

— Brian Michael Good

"If a quote does not fit the person's profile on social media or it sounds very familiar, look up the quote and tweet the quote correctly, honoring the author who took the time to write the quote that impacted your life."

— Brian Michael Good

"The pursuit of the American Dream is alive but not well and may seem obscure and improbable for most of us since is it is harder than ever to achieve with such an abundance of low paying jobs; but the truth is the American Dream has never been easy to attain. Yet, the elusive American Dream is still achievable for anyone with the right attitude, buying behavior, education, savings, knowing the value of hard work, and indomitable will."

— Brian Michael Good

"The truth about gossip is the misinformation that is created can influence a teenager or anyone else' decision to die by suicide. Gossip can kill someone emotionally, mentally, physically and spiritually"

— Brian Michael Good

"We have yet to explore the universe where there are estimated to be billions of Earth like planets. We might discover truths that would be inconceivable within our present day reality. Just because we have always hunted does not make it right to instill fear in the mammal we hunt."

— Brian Michael Good

"Only We-she-me-he – God – The Creator – Universe knows the truth."

— Brian Michael Good

"Mind control decays your ability to pursue and discover the truth. Mind control can use fear to control you. Do not let them control your free will with fear. Remove mind control and you will remove fear. Hit the reset button in your brain and live your life with less fear. Follow the truth but follow no one blindly."

— Brian Michael Good

"Be careful of anyone that states everything in a particular book or religion is one hundred percent the truth. There are over four thousand religions in our world and over thirty-four thousand Christian denominations. Only Weshemehe knows all the truth. Respect everyone's free will to search for the truth. Own your human gift of free will by exercising it; read, discover, assimilate, and question anything you want."

— Brian Michael Good

"I will not belong to a place of worship that says I have to believe one hundred percent in their dogma or their unique religious perspective. I refuse to give up my free will to pursue what I believe to be the truth."

— Brian Michael Good

What came first? The chicken or the egg?

The chicken came first. When a bird laid the first chicken egg; then the bird must have been a chicken because we called the first egg a chicken egg. Thus, the chicken came before the chicken egg. A chicken egg cannot be created without the development of a chicken embryo that starts in the chicken's oviducts.

Chickens always have, and chickens always will lay chicken eggs. Scientists have discovered that the egg cannot be produced without the protein ovocledidin-17 in the chicken's ovaries, so that means that the chicken must have come first. (For additional reading do a keyword search how scientists have solved the chicken and egg riddle.) Weshemehe gave the first chicken and the first turkey an Immaculate Conception. If We-she-me-he (God) gave Mary, the mother of Jesus Christ, an Immaculate Conception, then Weshemehe can give the first chicken an Immaculate Conception.

Chickens can have unfertilized eggs develop into embryos called parthenogenesis, chickens have had unfertilized eggs that developed into offspring including roosters. Get it, without the rooster. However, the roosters were born sickly and not as healthy as they normally would have been if the eggs were fertilized. The frequency of parthenogenesis in chicken eggs may be low but it does happen.

Parthenogenesis occurs in some chickens, turkeys, fish, and several kinds of insects, a few species of frogs, and lizards, including the Komodo dragon. The Komodo dragon lays unfertilized eggs that develop into hatched male Komodo Dragons.

"Parthenogenesis refers to the ability of unfertilized chicken and turkey eggs (and the eggs of other species) to develop embryos."

Parthenogenesis: Embryonic development in unfertilized eggs may affect normal fertilization and embryonic mortality." – Parthenogenesis, Wikipedia, the free encyclopedia

The human embryo (fetus) begin female for the first two weeks and only develops into a male embryo when the XY chromosome asserts itself and changes the genitalia from female to male.

This is why human males have breasts and nipples. The male sword is actually an enlarged woman's genitalia. ."

— Brian Michael Good

Excerpt from my book Never Surrender Your Soul

"your very essence"

Universal Values to Live By

Have tolerance and respect towards others and their culture.

No one should resolutely affect your pursuit of the truth.

Avoid judgment of ethnic, racial, sexual orientation, gender identity, and religious differences in society.

Do not attempt to control anyone's free will.

Avoid gossip, bullying, rumors, hearsay, hazing, harassment, shaming, shunning, and slurs.

Forgiving others sets us free.

Do not steal anything in any way.

Integrity and honor should be part of every fabric of your beliefs.

Do not kill emotionally, mentally, physically or spiritually.

Trust, faithfulness, and loyalty should define your relationships.

Value the passion you have for your life's work more than you value material gain.

Have kindness, compassion, and empathy towards others and the natural environment.

The number of people with no religion will continue to grow. You do not have to be religious to have good morals. "Universal Values to Live By" is meant to be a guide, a map for when we choose to use our free will and detour from the path we were taught to walk earlier in our lives. Free will is our greatest gift after life itself, that being said, free will must be exercised wisely, as much as humanly possible…

A person should weigh all twelve values equally, following one value and not another is as if you follow none of them. The true lesson gained from having good values comes from valuing the rights of others, not just your own.

When you meet another person or when two or more are gathered you will have the opportunity to create the gift of acceptance, the epitome of what humanity should be! The higher you raise yourself in the better treatment of others, the better view you will have of the future.

Humans have become more logical, facts build our knowledge and belief system. A logical person gathers facts and does not rely on faith alone. No one should resolutely affect your pursuit of the truth. We are gravitating towards building a belief system that is constructed mainly on materials based on facts. Without collaboration we could never make the strides of progress. No human is an island if they want to be successful.

Wealth

"I did not realize how much I had before my hurricanes occurred but each time after I weathered the storm. I wanted to live. There is always a possibility of a storm on the horizon. I hope that you too will find wisdom in these pearls that have washed ashore as a result of my hurricanes and count yourself a survivor."

— Brian Michael Good

"You do not get extra credit when you bequeath your wealth in your will because you cannot take money with you when you die."

— Brian Michael Good

"Authority, control, and wealth come with great responsibility. The Creator expects major shareholders, management and business owners to pay honest wages for an honest day's work. Greed does not give you any reward in the afterlife. You have already taken more than your fair share."

— Brian Michael Good

"There is enough wealth in our world to teach and share knowledge so each town or village can provide their own food, shelter, clothing and other commodities and services that are essential for survival."

— Brian Michael Good

"Luxuries are not a necessity and someday we will realize that the money spent on luxuries could have greatly influenced most of the world's problems."

— Brian Michael Good

"A person who chooses luxuries as prudently as they should choose their friendships will have a greater opportunity to be rewarded in the afterlife. Everything is a choice, enjoy life on Earth without a care in the world, or help others in need in the world."

— Brian Michael Good

"Now will be your defining moment. Will you look at giving away all your wealth as an empty glass, a glass half-full, or a glass half-empty? If you do this at the age of twenty-one, most likely your family paid for a great education which gave you the opportunity to make influential contacts. The other ninety-nine percent of your peers will never have the chance to make these connections. I hope that you will realize your glass is full without any money."

— Brian Michael Good

Wisdom

"There no better gift to another person than the gift of knowledge and understanding derived from wisdom."

— Brian Michael Good

"What you say does make a difference…

Think of this motto before you react or respond to any situation:

The 4 R's…Readiness, Respect, Right, and Reaction…"

— Brian Michael Good

"Today, I will try to stay in the eye of my hurricane where I am safe from the storm around me. I will try to deal with my hurricanes and struggles in life with no blame or excuses. But my hurricanes keep coming. I gain strength with each pearl of wisdom that washes ashore."

— Brian Michael Good

"A book is food for thought… By reading a well written book you will reap pearls of wisdom and have a lifetime of meals."

— Brian Michael Good

"Life's most valuable pearls of wisdom that are nourishment for the body, mind and soul are often found in quotes."

— Brian Michael Good

"A spiritual or personal growth self-help book can help you change your perspective allowing you to infuse new activities into your life."

— Brian Michael Good

"My hurricanes keep coming. I gain strength with each pearl of wisdom that washes ashore."

— Brian Michael Good

"Social, political, economic, and all rights should be equal to both women and men Women should have their turn to participate equally in running the planet. They did a better job until men took over thousands of years ago."

— Brian Michael Good

"We use the term human being very loosely in our society. I feel when we call someone a human being it should be a great compliment. A human is what you are but a human being is who you can become."

— Brian Michael Good

"Judaism, Hinduism, Christianity states that God is omnipresent; it might be referenced in Islam, Quran 2:115. If God is present everywhere (in all places at all times), then God is part of every atom in the universe. If the universe is God. Therefore, God does not have a gender.

If God does not have a gender, I choose to use the word Weshemehe (We-she-me-he), my own English name for God, who represents all genders. More importantly, it means more than just the male gender as the word God denotes to many of us. Weshemehe means we are all part of the universe and part of Weshemehe."

— Brian Michael Good

"I am in the eye of my hurricane where I am safe from the storm around me. I will try to deal with my hurricanes and struggles in life with no blame or excuses. Nevertheless, my hurricanes keep coming. I gain strength with each pearl of wisdom that washes ashore. We-she-me-he (the Creator) of second chances I am safe, for the moment at least."

— Brian Michael Good

Brian Michael Good Entrepreneur

Trademarks, Copyrighted Phrases, and Skincare Care Lines for

www.NutriCarePlus.com and www.TattooYouOrganics.com

Skin-Care and AfterCare that bring healing herbal nutrients and antioxidant A, C and E vitamins into the derma layer of skin.

"Capture the curative powers of NATURE!" ™

"The Road to a Better You!" ™

"Look Younger by Tomorrow" ™

"Now you too can enjoy the soothing and refreshing rejuvenation experience and have Skin that loves to be touched." ™

"First Aid Kit in a Bottle!" ™

"Take the Zing out of your Sting!" ™

"Take away Bottle!" ™

"Natural Body Care ™

Smooth Fusion ® Organics Skincare

Smooth Fusion ® Organics products for women and men are an advanced skin care line designed to heal problem skin conditions by using only natural and certified organic ingredients found in the herbal and organic tradition. Smooth Fusion ® Organics skin care line captures the curative powers of nature. We know that you will find these products to be effective, as our many customers already have!

Smooth Fusion ® Organics Antioxidant Serums, Organic Vegan Salves, and Organically Made Skin Regeneration Creams.

Balance of Nature ® Antioxidant Serum, from the Smooth Fusion ® Organics skin care line, has all the renowned ingredients which have been proven to slow down the aging process, minimize wrinkles and regenerate skin cells. This moisturizer floods your skin with essential fatty acids and vitamins and leaves your skin feeling extremely moist, soft and youthful.

BurniCure ® Antioxidant Serum and Quick Sunburn Relief is a highly effective organically made premium quality skincare product with organic and natural ingredients, paraben free, contains no harsh chemicals, is non-toxic with no heat. BurniCure restores the vitamins and fatty acids which re-hydrate the skin and bolsters the production of collagen and elastin with a unique regenerative effect.

BurniCure® Vegan is 100% Organic, Vegan, Antioxidant Serum and Quick Sunburn Relief.

BurniCare's ™ Eczema, Psoriasis Hives Salve from the Smooth Fusion line is comprised of 100% certified organic herbs & ingredients. This herbal salve will immediately begin to relieve itching and burning sensations brought on by these conditions and will rapidly reduce redness and inflammation of the skin.

Tattoo You ® Organics BurniCare ™ Organic Vegan AfterCare, Organic Vegan Salves, and SkinCare

----

Smooth Fusion ® Organics is a highly effective organically made premium quality skincare product with at least 80% certified organic ingredients and remaining ingredients are all natural, paraben free, contains no harsh chemicals, and is non-toxic with no heat. Our Organic salves and many of our antioxidant oils are 100% Certified Organic and cold pressed. Smooth Fusion ® Organics skincare restores the vitamins and fatty acids which re-hydrate the skin and bolsters the production of collagen and elastin with a unique regenerative effect.

Smooth Fusion ® Organics Skin Care formulas were developed from the consultation of Nutricare Plus™ Holistic Health Advisors. These Holistic Health Advisors have partnered with Nutricare Plus™ to bring you the exclusive Smooth Fusion ® Organics skin care line with herbal remedies that focus on specific health needs and overall wellness. Smooth Fusion products have been formulated by experienced licensed herbalists from around the country who have spent years studying conditions such as these and we are focused on bringing the finest herbal remedies that meet everyone's needs and surpass their expectations.

These herbal products are not found anywhere else. They have been tested on an open market for over twelve years with outstanding results; which is why we are bringing Smooth Fusion ®

Organics skincare products to you in far greater quantity than in 2003.

Nutricare Plus

Best Organic and Natural SkinCare Products

www.NutriCarePlus.com

Tattoo You Organics

Best Organic Vegan Tattoo, and Piercing AfterCare, and Skincare Products

www.TattooYouOrganics.com

Since 2001, *Nutricare Plus* and now *Tattoo You Organics* continue to market natural health and healing by offering special formulated skin care products, herbal remedies and pure emu oil for the body, mind, and spirit using only the highest quality of herbal, vegan, natural, and organic ingredients.

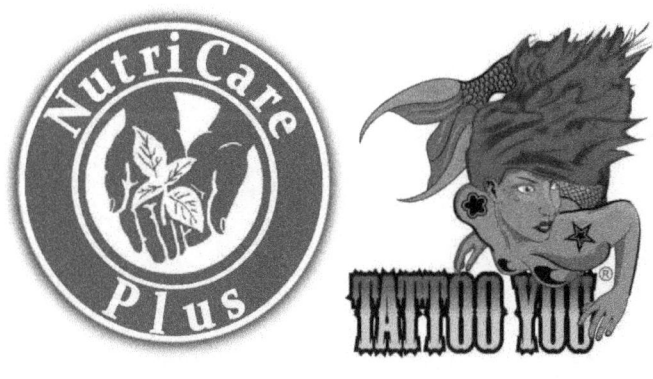

NutriCare Plus Testimonials

----

www.NutriCarePlus.com/Testimonials

Shirley Wood Testimonial

Esthetician to the Hollywood Stars

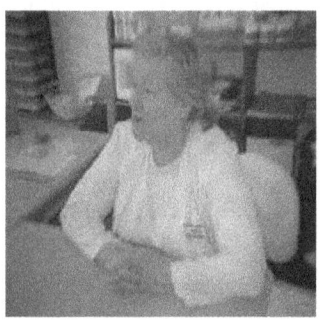

Shirley Wood

----

www.NutriCarePlus.com/Testimonials/Shirley-Wood-Esthetician-to-the-Hollywood-Stars

----

Ms. Wood for sixteen years was a staff Esthetician to the Hollywood stars while she was working for Warner Brothers in Burbank, CA consulting with makeup artists and hair stylists. She also was a consultant for prestigious salons in both Beverly Hills and Sherman Oaks, California where she provided esthetic consultation to many famous actors and actresses too numerous to mention.

Shirley Wood has spent her life's journey creating softer, firmer, younger looking faces.

"I tried the Nutricare Plus Emu oil followed by their antioxidant serum and antioxidant creams. After two weeks I was convinced that my skin had turned to satin. The derma layer had actually taken on a softer and smoother texture."

"I am certainly recommending the Nutricare Plus Pure Emu oil, antioxidant serum and antioxidant creams for skincare to all my clients in both Hollywood and throughout the world."

Now you too can enjoy the soothing and refreshing rejuvenation experience and have "Skin that loves to be touched" by Smooth Fusion ®.

----

www.NutriCarePlus.com/face-creams-serums

Robin Ball Testimonial

Licensed Esthetician, Medical Assistant, Consultant

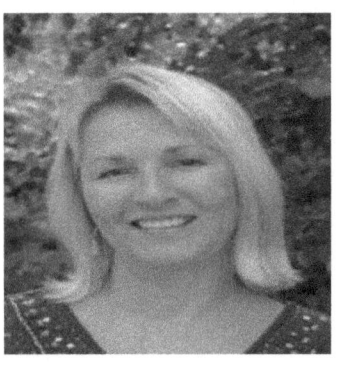

Robin Ball

----

www.NutriCarePlus.com/Testimonials/Robin-Ball-Licensed-Esthetician-Medical-Assistant-Consultant

----

"I blend the two products together on my fingertips to make a cocktail moisturizer and my skin looks and feels great! My client's and I love these products! They will keep your skin looking younger without paying enormous prices. "I recommend these products to everyone wanting smoother younger looking skin and wrinkle reduction."

"As a professional Licensed Esthetician and Medical Assistant, I have used many quality skincare lines over the past seven years. I discovered Triple Refined Pure Emu Oil after seeing it on Oprah and found it to be the most intense moisturizer I have ever used. Then I found Nutricare Plus Pure Emu Oil which is exactly the same Pure Emu Oil "seen on Oprah" but at a fraction of the cost!"

----

www.NutriCarePlus.com/face-creams-serums

Peaceful Worlds

----

www.Facebook.com/PeacefulWorlds

"Striving for a more Peaceful World, one human at a time."

Peaceful Worlds is a 501(c)(3) not-for-profit organization whose goal is to be an outreach initiative providing answers, information, and provide resources for a more Peaceful World on Earth, our Solar System, and the estimated hundred billion Galaxies in the Universe.

Take the "Peaceful Worlds Lemon-Aid Challenge.

We need to talk about lemons, in other words, help create a more Peaceful World by disengaging from mankind's terror. Take the I am Peace… We are Peace... Pledge. We would like you to take the #PeacefulWorldsLemonAidChallenge as a way to raise money for the Peaceful Worlds non-profit. We challenge you to eat three slices of lemon or donate $10.00 to Peaceful Worlds.

Donate to Peaceful Worlds, Non-Profit and tweet your support at" #PeacefulWorldsLemonAidChallenge

----

"When life gives you lemons, make lemonade" is a proverbial phrase used to encourage optimism and a can-do attitude in the face of adversity or misfortune. Lemons suggest bitterness, while lemonade is a sweet drink.– Wikipedia

----

Never Surrender to Mankind's Terror, Be a Survivor, SURVIVE one day at a time knowing that no one can defeat the human race. The human race can only defeat themselves.

Best To Live

"You are not alone and you are not forgotten."

Best to Live, is a 501(c)(3) non-profit, whose goal is to be an outreach initiative providing answers, information, and provide resources for health needs and overall wellness for anyone who needs to survive emotional, mental, or physical stress.

We hope anyone who has been exposed to violence, abuse, extreme stress, or loss of an important person will seek us out if you need a friend to lean on.

The *Best to Live* logo has the Seed of Life symbol behind the text. The blue hues indicate willingness to see solutions in everything.

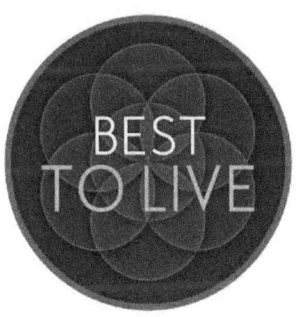

www.BestToLive.org

Never Surrender, Be a Survivor, SURVIVE one day at a time knowing that it is Best to Live

*Take the "**Best to Live LemonAid Challenge**" to Help Stop Self-Harm*

We need to talk about lemons in other words, Help Stop Self-Harm. We would like you to take the "LemonAid Challenge" as a way to raise money for the *Best to Live* Non-Profit. We challenge you to eat three slices of lemon or donate $10.00 to *Best To Live*.

----

http://www.Besttolive.org/Donate.html

----

aid alone anyone best
besttolive challenge cutting
dollars donate donatetenusd
donatetobesttolive eat eighty
forgotten harm help hopes
involves lemon
lemonaidchallenge live
money needs non-profit object
percent provide raise self self-
harm sharp skin slices stabbing
stop stop-self-harm stress support taking talk
wedges

Donate to Best To Live, Non-Profit and tweet your support at" #B2LLemonAidCHL "

"When life gives you lemons, make lemonade" is a proverbial phrase used to encourage optimism and a can-do attitude in the face of adversity or misfortune. Lemons suggest bitterness, while lemonade is a sweet drink."

– When life gives you lemons, make lemonade, From Wikipedia, the free encyclopedia

Eighty percent of self-harm involves stabbing or cutting the skin with a sharp object. By taking the "LemonAid Challenge," we can show our support for anyone who self-harms by eating three slices of lemon. This will show that they are not Alone or Forgotten, in the hopes that they will eat a few wedges of lemon before they Self-Harm, hoping they will forget why they were about to cut themselves.

Social Media Links

Brian Michael Good

Author | Spearhead Thinker | Peace Advocate |

Entrepreneur | Genius | Precious Savant

Meet the Author: www.BrianMichaelGood.com

Twitter: www.twitter.com/1PearlofWisdom

Facebook: www.facebook.com/BrianMichaelGood

LinkedIn: www.linkedin.com/in/Brian-Michael-Good-9a43a0a9

Peaceful Worlds, a 501(c)(3) not-for-profit

Facebook: https://www.facebook.com/PeacefulWorlds

Website: www.PeacefulWorlds.org (coming soon)

Best to Live Foundation, a 501(c)(3) not-for-profit

Website: www.BestToLive.org

Twitter: www.twitter.com/Best2Live

Facebook: www.facebook.com/Best2Live

Spiritual and Personal Growth Self-Help Books

Facebook: www.facebook.com/BrianMichaelGoodauthor

Tattoo You Organics

Organic Herbal Infused Vegan Tattoo, Piercing,

and Skincare Products

Website: www.TattooYouOrganics.com

Twitter: www.twitter.com/TatUAftercare

Facebook: www.facebook.com/TattooYouOrganics

Pinterest: www.pinterest.com/TatUAfterCare

Instagram: www.instagram.com/TatUAfterCare

NutriCare Plus

Best Organic and Natural Skincare Products

Website: www.NutriCarePlus.com

NutriCare Plus Shop: www.NutriCarepPlus.com/shop.html

Twitter: www.twitter.com/NCPCARES

Facebook: www.facebook.com/NutriCarePlus

Pinterest: www.pinterest.com/NutriCarePlus

Instagram: www.instagram.com/NutriCarePlus

The Green Postal Store

Facebook: www.facebook.com/The-Green-Postal-Store-699395376867357

Thank You

No person is an island if they want to succeed. I would like to thank the following people who helped me through my journey of writing:

- Helga Holscher who I met in 2008 and who reviewed my journal in early 2009 gave me much needed encouragement.

- Stacie Morgan, even though she was working on her novel in the research stage, reviewed my writings and gave me suggestions that helped me to begin to pull together some initial ideas that proved helpful in the creation of the book's vision in 2010.

- Bryan Hunt, a great talent, who I would like to recognize for his strong work ethic. Bryan has a college degree in Animation. He helped me over several years with my passion for organic and natural skincare by creating the numerous labels, brochures and advertising I needed created. His expertise certainly helped keep my hope alive.

- I would like to thank Laurie Callihan, Dara Rochlin, Christine Rice, and Charlene Truxler who assisted me in the editing and formatting process during various stages of "Never Surrender Your Soul", "RESET: Control, Alt, Delete", "Quotes Of Wisdom To Live By", and "World Peace, Peaceful Worlds, Game Over".

- In addition, I would like to thank Shelter, Inc. Cambridge, Massachusetts, HomeStart, Inc., Cambridge, Massachusetts, and the Waterfront Rescue Mission, Pensacola, Florida for providing a roof over my head when I was a person of need.

Book Offer

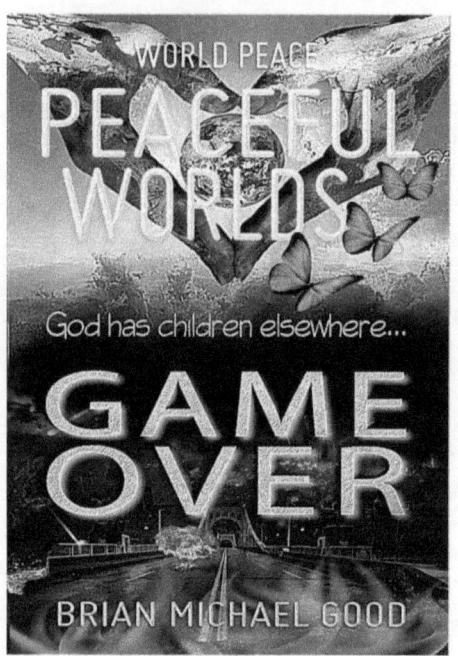

World Peace, Peaceful Worlds, Game Over

Here is the link to visit the book page:

www.authl.it/ B01JUR29UW?d

The human race is on the cusp of either taking more strategic steps towards a more Peaceful World and eventually World Peace or Game Over — Armageddon.

Ask yourself this… What would you do for World Peace if you knew the end was near? Game Over — End of the World?

The future; a more Peaceful World — Peaceful Worlds can only be changed in the present. Free will, a human's greatest gift after life itself comes with a price. God will not save you. The human race (women) must save themselves. You may be the missing link that is the difference between a more Peaceful World... World Peace... or a highly probable World War III — Game Over — Apocalypse...

What are you waiting for? The clocks ticking...

Oh... It's a nuclear clock.

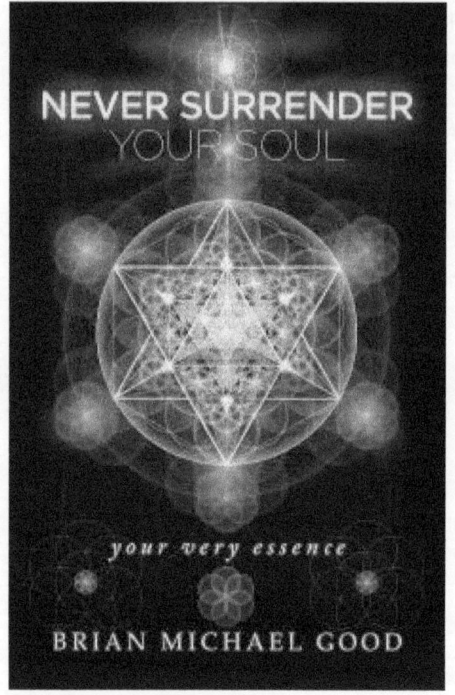

Never Surrender Your Soul – your very essence

Here is the link to visit the book page:

www.authl.it/0986252794?d

If you wish for personal – spiritual growth and fulfillment in your life and less fear, it is possible! Never Surrender Your Soul unlike other self-help books is written specifically to help you to find the encouragement, strength, and spiritual growth that you will need to change your perspective with less mind control so you can live a hopeful life that creates a path with less fear.

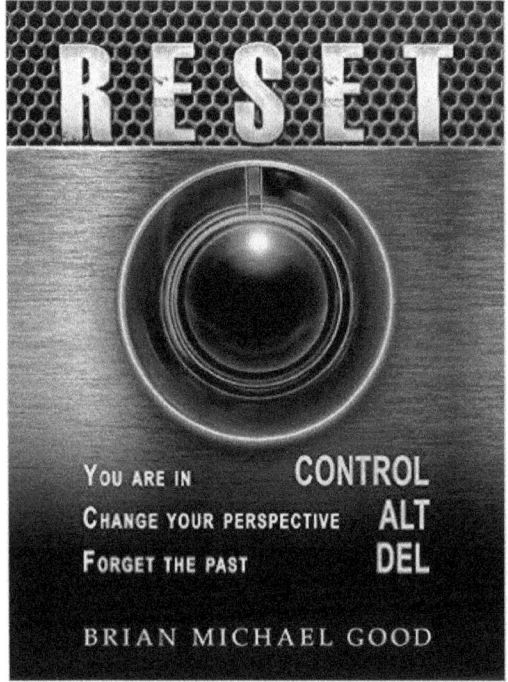

RESET: Control, Alt, Delete

Here is the link to visit the book page:

www.authl.it/ 098625276X?d

Learn how to rise from the ashes of defeat. Get self-help, Embrace positive thinking, Live a happier life, and Find your destiny.

RESET: Control, Alt, Delete, unlike other self-help books, is written specifically to help you to find the encouragement, strength, and personal growth that you will need to change your perspective with positive thinking so you can live a hopeful life that creates a path allowing you to find your destiny.

No one can defeat you; you can only defeat yourself. No one can truly save you. You must save yourself. The question is what are you willing to do to change your life? There is hope and a way out! Help yourself by reading Never Surrender Your Soul, RESET: Control, Alt, Delete, and Quotes of Wisdom to Live By find answers and change your life for the better.

Take action by getting yourself a copy of one of Brian's four books. You will be so happy you did!

Join our email list

----

www.BrianMichaelGood.com/contact-me

Write a Review

----

http://amzn.to/2cwW1qU

It will have an impact and you can make a difference.

BRIAN MICHAEL GOOD

Lightning Source UK Ltd.
Milton Keynes UK
UKHW011825230522
403389UK00001B/209